Fabulously
You
Book Two

Fabulously You
Book Two

Feel Amazing
& Thrive

Pamela Sommers

COPYRIGHT

Edited by Diana McMahon Collis

First Edition

Print ISBN: 978-1-9163587-4-4

Hardcover ISBN: 978-1-9163587-5-1

Epub ISBN: 978-1-9163587-2-0

omissions, whether such errors or omissions result from accident, negligence, or any other cause.

This represents general information only. Before making any financial or investment decisions, we recommend you consult a financial planner to take into account your personal investment objectives, financial situation and individual needs.

General

This book is designed to provide information and motivation to the reader. It is sold with the understanding that the author is not engaged to render any type of psychological, legal, or any other kind of professional advice. The content of each article is the sole expression and opinion of its author. No warranties or guarantees are expressed or implied by the author's choice to include any of the content in this volume. The individual author shall not be liable for any physical, psychological, emotional, financial, or commercial damages, including, but not limited to, special, incidental, consequential or other damages. Please be advised that you are responsible for your own choices, actions, and results.

I dedicate this book to all the women in my life,

including my friends & family.

Thank you for your continued love, support and friendship.

May your life be filled with blessings and abundance

as you continue to be fabulous.

CONTENTS

INTRODUCTION

What is it that you really want from life? Are you content with your life as it is? Is there a part of you that wants more out of it? I imagine that there's more to you than meets the eye! If you know this to be true, then what are you waiting for? Have you been imagining that you'll just wait for things to fall into your lap, and then smile sweetly and say, 'Thank you'? Or are you ready to make things happen and be the gamechanger of your own world? Will you be content with only observing the success of others from afar, or would you prefer to play the starring role in your own life story?

I dare you to challenge yourself by being the person you've always dreamt of being! The chances are that you've got what it takes, already; you just don't know it yet.

Feel Amazing and Thrive is the second book of the *Fabulously You* series. It can be read in conjunction with the first book, *Live A Life You*

Love, or as a standalone volume. It is for women at the prime of their lives, who want to live life their way, without limitations — and with no permission required from others.

This book is like pure dynamite! It will get you to explore the deepest part of yourself– a possibly uncomfortable, but necessary, process – in order for you to shift whatever's been holding you back. It will help reveal your inner superhero. Why sit back and watch others, when you can be that woman of wonder? It's time for you to rise up and take back the reins!

By the time you have finished reading this book, you will feel revived and raring to go, with a fresh outlook on life and newfound sparkle in your eye. With your passion reignited, nothing can hold you back. You will be ready to soar!

Watch out world; there's a brand-new hero in town, and femininity is her superpower!

Are you ready?

CHAPTER 1

Courage

It takes courage

It takes a great deal of courage to do many things in life and this applies to both small and large undertakings. A specific, personal context may make the process harder, sometimes. We each have our own challenges to respect. For someone who suffers with anxiety, for instance, going out into a crowded environment takes a great deal of courage. For anyone who has been used to the freedom of their own space, making a life-changing commitment to a relationship can require enormous bravery. Courage comes in many forms and can also affect people in different ways. While one person won't think twice about being the first to get up and dance at a party, another may require some Dutch courage before deciding to make a move.

If you're feeling depressed, or going through a tragic upheaval, just getting out of bed in the morning can require courage. This is not all 'black and white'; there are plentiful shades of grey in between, too.

Courage requires both energy and enthusiasm to grow; without an initial, strong intention, there is little chance of moving forward. But how can you get from where you are, to where you want to be? This is something that can take time, patience and a little friendly persuasion. All right – even a lot of persuasion! It can, nevertheless, be done.

To explore how it might work, in reality, let's use the scenario of going outside, after a long period of time.

Baby steps

It helps to remember that you don't have to go 'all in', straight away. We can, of course, sometimes leap into an activity fully and get great results. But there may be the risk of an experience putting us off for life, if we try to do too much too soon. If, instead, you can take things slowly, and go at a steady pace, you're more likely be consistent in what you manage to do. You're also more likely to repeat the new task, as opposed to making it a 'one-off'. Here's a practical suggestion for if you've been at home for ages. As you may be feeling a little apprehensive about going out and being surrounded by lots of people, why not go to a place close by, to begin with? Then try somewhere further away.

Short time

You don't have to go out for all of the day, or night, either. Try, instead, going out for just an hour or two and seeing how you feel. You'll probably be surprised at how quickly a couple of hours can go by!

It gets easier

The main thing to remember is that the more often you do something, the easier it becomes. Eventually, you'll be able to reach a point when it hardly crosses your mind as a problem, and then you can go out effortlessly– at just a moment's notice.

Have company

You don't have to do everything alone, to demonstrate courage. There are no rule books about this. There is no harm, for example, in going out with a friend, or with someone close who understands you. It may well be more pleasant, because it takes the pressure off, and you can chat with one another. Company can be a very good thing – as long as it's the right kind of company, of course. It's often nicer to hang around with positive people, who look for the good in others – as opposed to people who tend to be critical in their attitudes.

Other people's actions

One thing that can save a lot of unnecessary stress and time is the realisation that, no matter how hard you try, you can't control how other people act or behave. You can, however, control how you react – and how you feel about what others are saying or doing. While this isn't always easy, as with many things, a little practice goes a long way.

Pep talk

One way of working on your own reactions is by giving yourself a little pep talk! You can include affirmations to go with it. Although this may sound silly at first, my suggestion is to give it a go and just see how you get on.

Make a habit, every morning, of looking at yourself in the mirror — not in a negative, fault-finding way, but in a loving, 'You're amazing!' way. Say to yourself, 'I am an amazing, lovely, human being.' Then, continue with, 'I make friends easily' and 'I am surrounded by kind and positive people, everywhere I go'. Finish off by telling yourself how wonderful you are, mentioning at least three qualities about yourself.

Try to say these to yourself every morning, as well as before you go out. This will help train your mind to expect good things to happen around you. Most of all, it will help you to feel better about yourself.

Patience

Don't worry if things don't always go to plan; just get up and try again! Very few things that are worth having are achieved instantly. Be gentle with yourself. Remember, you have come a long way. Given time and patience, things will fall into place.

Finding courage in the everyday

Courage doesn't have to involve doing something extreme, such as climbing a mountain, or sky diving. It could relate to walking into a restaurant that you've never been to before, and sitting down by yourself to have a meal. Or asking someone you've liked for ages out for a coffee.

Look at the little situations in your life that remind you of where it has taken courage for you to do something. For instance, maybe you voiced your opinion at a staff meeting, when you would normally have kept quiet. Or perhaps you stood up for a passenger on a bus, whom you felt was being mistreated. All these things take courage. Like most things in life, the more often you do them, the easier it gets to find that courage.

Don't wait until tomorrow to be courageous. Practise it today and see how it goes! Notice the way you feel. You might well find out how brave you are, after all. Your courage just needed a little persuasion, to come out.

Enthusiasm

Once you've overcome your first few hurdles, you'll have gained the courage to try new things. As your newfound confidence begins to grow, so too will your appetite for bigger and brighter experiences. Before you know it, your eagerness will know no bounds. You'll be raring to go, with an unfaltering enthusiasm for life!

You can do it

Having a 'can do' approach to life is a shortcut to creating success. When you feel good, you're likely to have more courage to do the things you want to do. This is a winning formula!

CHAPTER 2

It's all in the mind

Your mindset

Mindset is how most things start. First you begin with a thought, then you perhaps talk about it. Eventually, there comes a point where you need to take action to see it through.

You may have heard someone say that it's 'all in your head', or 'all in the mind', particularly if they're talking about someone complaining about physical ailments. The truth is that the mind is an incredible masterpiece. Similar to computers, our brains are made up of many components and intricacies that are complex, yet necessary for us to perform even the simplest daily tasks. Not only does your brain store memory; it can also regulate hormones, supply oxygen, pump blood throughout your body and enable you to move by way of motor skills. Although your mind has been

29

used to thinking certain ways since your birth, it also has the ability to be re-programmed into forming better habits – in a way that can benefit you immensely.

As a qualified NLP practitioner, I am familiar in the ways of – if you like – 'commanding' the mind, to help guide anyone into a more positive mindset.

Everything you do begins with mindset. For instance, when you first get up in the morning, your thoughts govern what type of day you will have, even before you have stepped out of bed! Just notice: do you wake up raring to get on with the day, full of excitement as to what lies ahead? Or have you already made up your mind that it's going to be another mundane day, where you have to just get through?

How you feel first thing in the morning can have a huge impact on your day. Even if you have got out of the 'wrong side' of the bed, though, things don't have to remain that way. You can change your feelings, by simply deciding that you are going to have a great day – and then act accordingly! Once you have made this decision, just act as though you mean it – and watch how your energy levels begin to soar. Suddenly, what you would have first found to be a mission, you can now do with ease – and things will start to go more smoothly.

For example, let's say you spill some milk on the floor; you can simply clean it up and put it down to being 'one of those things'. There's no need to make a big deal about it. If you are caught up in traffic while driving, you can simply start humming along to a song on the radio, or choose to listen to an uplifting podcast. Setting yourself up to have a positive day can work wonders for your mood, taking you to a point where you start to find joy in what you do.

Rollercoaster

I learnt the importance of mindset when I became an entrepreneur – although, admittedly, I wasn't quite prepared for the rollercoaster life that went with it! Not many people talk about this aspect; they tend to focus more on the money-making side of things. Boy, did it take me by surprise! First of all, I just assumed that everyone would support me and be there for me if I needed them, appreciating my determination to succeed. On speaking to other entrepreneurs, I discovered quite quickly that my assumption couldn't have been further from the truth. Many of them had unsupportive family and friends. Whilst the entrepreneurs were celebrating building their first websites, or posting their first blogs, others around them couldn't see what all the fuss was about. It is a shock to find out that friends, family or perhaps people you've known for a lifetime – are not as excited about your latest launch as you'd hoped they would be. This is when mindset steps in. You have to develop a pretty thick skin quite fast and get to the point where you know it doesn't matter if others don't see the value in what you're doing. That it's okay for them to have their opinion, or a lack of interest, because they're living life their way, not yours. You have to back yourself to realise your potential, regardless what others think of you and what you're doing. Remember that, for every person who is not 'for' you, there are at least five people

who are, or will be, rooting for you and who
will love you no matter what. Focus on them!

Train your mind

You have to train your mind to think
positively, even when surrounded by a world
of negativity. It's not easy! If it was, then
everyone else would be doing the same thing.
But it is possible. Not everyone is born to
lead, either. It takes a special kind of person to
think big and dream bigger. While others say
'You can't do that', encourage yourself to
think outside the box and find a way that you
can get around any problem. More often than
not, you'll find a way – at least if you want it
badly enough!

Remember the reason

One of the things that helps me is to
remember the reason why I started my
entrepreneurial life in the first place. When
you feel you are at your lowest point, ask
yourself the same. Your reason will help see
you through and drive you forward. At times
when you think nothing is going right, your
reason will keep you going and remind you of

33

your strengths. A strong mind can carry you through the toughest journey. Look after it; strengthen and nurture it and you will reap the benefits.

Do things to help you stay in a positive frame of mind. Exercise is great, for instance, for helping keep focused. It will clear your head and provide a terrific stress-release. Eating and drinking healthily can also help you with energy levels. Good quality sleep can provide a sense of well-being and is great for maintaining mental alertness. I have found that regularly praying, meditating, saying affirmations and doing visualisations can also assist in keeping a successful mindset. It is important, as well, to celebrate your wins and have gratitude for all the lovely things you have in your life. This attracts more good things into your life. These activities will all help keep you prepared for success and make you feel you can achieve whatever you put your mind to.

Choose positivity! This is so important because, if you have a successful mindset, you're far more likely to achieve your goals and dreams. You will also inspire others around you, along the way.

Mindset is a tool that can take you from where you are now to where you want to go. Use it wisely and it can set you free to be the person you are truly meant to be.

CHAPTER 3

By yourself

Don't wait for others

There's no need to wait for others before you
go somewhere or do something, because you
could be waiting a very long time – or,
indeed, never. A lot of people appear too
afraid to venture out by themselves, or start
anything fun, even if it's something they've
always wanted to do. They tend to feel safer
and more confident if someone is there with
them, by their side, as if holding their hand. I
understand this concept completely. Even so,
there may come a point in life when you need
to gather up the gumption inside you and just
do what you have always wanted to do,
regardless of whether you have company or
not. Besides, it's your life – and you have the
greatest know how on leading it in the best
way for you.

Be self-sufficient

Luckily, this has never been a problem for me, since I have always been – or shall we say *had* to be – self-sufficient. This has served me well, in a way, teaching me to be independent. I used to see being self-sufficient as a bad thing, especially when I was at school. I noticed other girls in small groups, laughing and chatting, while I was observing from a distance or had only one or two friends. I remember asking my teacher about why I was never included in those groups. She said she was surprised I felt the way I did, because I had always been regarded as self-sufficient. She meant that I didn't seem to require anyone else be around me. I now take that as a compliment! It has helped reinforce my belief that you do not need anyone else to do the things you, yourself, love and feel good about. That's right—there's no permission required!

Have fun

This theme was quite an eye-opener for me and has since served me well on numerous occasions in life. I recall, for instance, when I was eighteen and renting a room in shared accommodation. I felt a strong urge to go clubbing one Wednesday evening. I phoned around, asking a couple of friends if they would like to join me, but nobody wanted to. So, I decided I had two options; I could either stay at home and feel lonely and frustrated, or venture out by myself and have some fun. Guess what I did? Yes, my playful and possibly slightly rebellious side took hold of me – and out I went! I remember getting on the tube to Piccadilly Circus in London and walking along, in search of a club to go to. I felt the excitement in the air and was pleasantly pleased to see many people out and about, just like me, ready to party and enjoy the fun. I loved that it was dark and filled with brightly coloured lights. I felt like a kid who was wide awake when she was supposed to be asleep – full of mischief and ready to go! I soon met and chatted to various people, just by walking along the street. Then I encountered an Italian guy, who said he was tired, and asked me to go somewhere quiet with him instead of clubbing. I politely declined, saying I couldn't – and that I just had to dance. I could feel the energy racing

FABULOUSLY YOU: FEEL AMAZING & THRIVE

through me, which needed to be expressed through dance. I loved to dance; it took me to another world. It's a world where magic happens and where you can be anything you want to be. So, I entered a club and got my wish.

I had such a wonderful night! I didn't drink alcohol – I never did when I went clubbing, because I liked to feel in control of my mind and my body, especially if I was out alone. I was very sensible and aware of safety, which enabled me to enjoy myself in a safe environment without any worry, and ensure I got home safely.

Keep a sense of adventure

There was another occasion, in my thirties, when I decided to go away alone, to have some quality 'me' time and enjoy myself. I booked a trip to Sweden, as it was on my 'to-go' list, of places to visit. I was working as a manager in a bank back then and a friend and colleague was concerned for me, even though she almost always travelled by herself. She asked if I would call her regularly from Sweden, else she would worry; so, I agreed and did so. I felt like I was going on an adventure! It was exciting and had an element of surprise which got my adrenaline rushing. I made so many friends, simply by walking along the street. I have noticed this hardly ever happens when with other people. Being by yourself, makes you instantly more approachable! I remember one guy, from the USA, who had a guitar attached to his back; he said he thought I was so brave and cool, travelling by myself. I began to see a pattern emerge, where others also thought I was cool. This was quite a revelation to me, as it had been a long time since I was called 'cool'. I found I never felt alone while I was away. I made so many friends, it was virtually impossible to do so. I returned back to England feeling excited, energised and empowered. I felt I had discovered something about myself that I had never known – or had perhaps forgotten. I realised how strong I was and how I was able to take risks; this was a side of me that I hardly ever showed, usually.

There's no pressure

I realise that times were different back then. It was okay to go places without worrying too much. There seems to be more crime around these days. I will emphasise, therefore, that I'm not saying that you have to go out at night by yourself. What I am saying is that you don't need to wait for others to join you, to have a good time – nor to do the things you've always wanted to do. I've been to the cinema by myself and even dined out by myself. At first, I was worried about others' thinking, e.g., 'there's the saddo, by herself'. But, once I started chatting and getting to know others, I found it wasn't that bad. I'd go as far to say it was quite fun, in fact! There are definite benefits. For instance, if you're dining alone you can eat as much or as little as you like, of whatever you like. You don't have to worry about how you look. The pressure is off and you can make friends along the way, which would hardly ever happen if you were with another person, or in a group.

Although I can be a bit of a loner, I still love chatting and laughing with other people.

Whether you are with others, or more of a loner, remember: you're cool!

CHAPTER 4

Live in alignment

Stay aligned

Live your life in a way that feels completely right for you. When you are aligned with everything you say and do, you'll feel more content within yourself. Sometimes this is easier said than done, especially when the pressure is on. That might be when you are trying to land the client of your dreams and are willing to do almost anything to persuade them to say yes, even if it means sacrificing what you hold dear to you. This can include your time and other things you value greatly. It's always a good idea to take a moment to pause in situations like these. Pausing gives you options and may just save you from actions you'll regret.

This won't seem easy at first, especially if you're used to giving unconditionally, with little in return. But, like most things, the more you practise, the easier it'll become. Firstly, you need to get familiar with what your values are, considering what matters to you the most. A good way to find this out is by journaling.

What is important to you?

Ask yourself, 'What is important to me?' and take some time to really home in on the answer. Think about the 'non-negotiables' in your life. We all have these, although sometimes we let them slip by, without a moment's thought. We may then wonder why we feel so resentful; almost like something has been taken from us without permission. Does this sound familiar? Part of it will be because we haven't made them a priority, or even identified what they are. So, what is it you value the most? It could be your time and how you spend it. Personally, I like to keep Sundays free for spending quality time with my family, as well as recuperation time for me. My Sunday is a time when I get to rest and recharge, in preparation for the week ahead. I have found that if I don't have this time, or it gets disturbed for some reason, the effect spills out onto the rest of the week – and things may not go quite according to plan.

Another example relates to someone I know, who likes to read for half an hour before going to bed. If they get interrupted, or something comes up, and they don't get their reading time, they find their sleep gets disturbed – and then they become quite grouchy the next day.

Prioritise what matters

Once you have found out what's important to you, focus on making it a priority –and build your days and weeks around it. I know this may sound strange at first, especially if you're not used to placing your needs above others. But you'll soon discover how this one transition can affect everything you do – and the way you do it – in a very positive way. It can impact other people around you too, including your nearest and dearest. Give it a go; you'll be amazed at the difference it brings to you all and how much more contented you feel!

Get comfortable

Now that you know what you hold closest to your heart, you'll need to practise getting comfortable with creating boundaries around this. If, for instance, you want to make sleep a priority, turning your mobile phone off by a certain time each evening will mean you won't be disturbed; distractions will be kept to a minimum. Taking control like this will help to develop confidence. It will show that you are putting yourself first and valuing what is important to you.

Value your worth

If you are an entrepreneur – as a specific example – you may want to charge a certain price for your product or programme, because you know how much time and effort you have taken into putting it out into the world. This can be tough, especially if you're used to trying to please people; you may feel bad about charging the full price for something. But how about valuing yourself, too?

Entrepreneur or otherwise, you are just as valuable as the next person. You deserve to live a life full of love, happiness and abundance, too. You also deserve to be paid for your time, services or products. By charging your worth, you are not taking worth away from anyone else. Read that again:

By charging your worth, you are not taking worth away from anyone else

When you discount something heavily, or are virtually giving it away – because you feel you ought to – you are subconsciously saying to the Universe, 'That's okay; it's only me'. This almost implies that you don't matter. This, in turn, can bring up other limiting beliefs, such as you're not good enough, or not worthy, catch my drift? And before you know it, if this attitude goes unchecked, it can become a self-fulfilling prophecy, whereby if you don't feel your service or product is good enough, then – guess what – no one else will do, either. If you can't feel aligned and believe in yourself, then why should they?

The same applies if you yearn to live in a more pleasant environment. Perhaps you'd love a nicer home with beautiful surroundings. Start by appreciating and valuing yourself, then work on putting changes into place. You might, for example, clean, declutter and tidy your space until it is in keeping with how you want to feel. It will then become a place that nourishes your soul – and a home that you are happy to be in. This all helps with living in alignment.

So, put your hand on your heart right now and say to yourself, out loud, 'I am worthy. I am good enough. I deserve to live a life full of love, happiness and abundance'. Repeat this three times and do it regularly, until you truly believe it – from the bottom of your heart. When you start believing in yourself and what you do, others will, also.

Get in tune with yourself

If you are familiar with getting in tune with yourself and listening to your inner guidance, that's wonderful. Doing so enables you to tap in and connect with yourself in a deeper way. If you're exploring this, here's an exercise you can try, to help you get familiar with self-connection and listening to your inner voice:

CHAPTER 4: LIVE IN ALIGNMENT

- Say two statements to yourself, which you know to be true or false (i.e. to which your body would give 'yes' or 'no' signals as answers) and then watch for where any changes occur in your body. For example, say to yourself, 'My name is [insert your name]', then say out loud, 'Yes', and repeat your name. See how your body responds to this positive, 'Yes' response.

- Then say to yourself, 'My name is [insert someone else's name]'. As this is false information, your body is likely to give a negative or, 'No' response. Take a moment to notice the feeling you get and where in the body this occurs.

- Observe the difference between your feelings and the way your body responds to both statements. This is how to test your natural alignment either towards or away from something. You may even find your body moves forward towards your positive, 'Yes' response and physically

51

moves back or away when you say your negative, 'No' response.

So, the next time someone asks you to commit to something and you feel uncomfortable about it, but can't quite put your finger on why, remember this exercise. It will help you tune into what feels right to you. The more you do this, the more confidence you will have in trusting your own inner compass.

Live in alignment

Now that you are getting to know yourself at a deeper level, it will become easier to stay aligned with what feels right. Remember, when something doesn't *feel* right, the chances are it really isn't right for you – or at least not at this moment in time. Be discerning and stay true to your heart, for your heart seldom misleads you. If you can live in alignment with your soul, the chances are, you'll feel much happier for it.

CHAPTER 5

Appreciate yourself

What do you secretly long for?

Are you fulfilled? Is there a feeling from deep within you, perhaps something you've been wanting, or even aching to do? But, possibly, due to the demands of everyday life, those plans have fallen by the wayside – or, worse still – have been lost, almost forgotten, buried under mounds of things on your to-do list. Maybe the to-do list seems more important. Is that really the case? Or is it that you don't care to admit to yourself that you maybe don't feel you are worthy enough to make your dreams happen? Perhaps you think it's okay for others, and you are happy to stand aside and watch, while others bask in the limelight.

You may try to deny it, or skirt around the issue, but I suspect there is more to you than meets the eye. I imagine you have a true vision and I see myself standing beside you, watching how you secretly long for greener pastures, or streets paved in gold. How am I so convinced? Because I once stood where you are now. I used to stand in the shadows while my best friend grabbed the limelight. I would look down to the floor if someone called my name, for fear of overstepping the mark. I literally used to 'keep my head down and get on with it', desperate to keep a low profile.

Dream of fairy tales

The reality of how things were, for me, couldn't have been more opposite. While I played a supportive role to my friend, there was a part of me that secretly ached for my own success. I used to dream of being in fairy tales and playing the lead role. In school plays, I not only knew all the lines of the lead female character, but also knew every single word for all the other characters in the play! I recall one day when the lead female couldn't act, for some reason. The teacher asked if anyone else knew her part. I was desperate to put my hand up and say, 'Yes, I do', but I looked down to the floor, instead. By the time

I raised my head again, I was watching the opportunity that had just been within my reach disappear. I remember feeling intense frustration and annoyance at myself, for not having the courage to go after what I wanted. I just let it slip out of my grasp. I remember the sadness I felt that others would never know how talented I actually was. But even worse, that the reason for this was because I didn't show up for myself.

Show up for yourself

I'm sure there are many times where you haven't shown up for yourself. Sometimes it's easier to stand up for others than to fend for yourself. Many of us feel that others deserve to be supported – but what about you? It's time, now, to start valuing yourself for the wonderful person that you are! Start counting the many blessings of you. Focus on all the beautiful things you do, every day. Build upon your qualities, including the ones you keep hidden from others. You deserve more than the mundane. You deserve to be lavished with love and cared for.

So, decide to show up for yourself, once in a while. Take pride and enjoy sharing all you have to offer. Give yourself space to blossom into the wonderful human being you are meant to be. I can see you bloom! It's now your turn to fulfil these promises to yourself. Now is the time for you to flourish.

Tap into your heart

Tap into your heart and listen to its inner guidance. We all have that inner voice; it's just that some choose to listen to it more than others. Try it and see. Give yourself ten minutes of quiet time a day. Go to a place where you can't be disturbed. Close your eyes, if it helps. Sometimes, I place the palm of my hand on my heart area and just feel it and listen to my heart beat. Try it yourself. This is you, truly tapping into your heart. Now, listen…what can you hear? What is your heart telling you?

It may take a while to get into the zone and tune into how you are feeling, but, the more you do so, the easier it will get. Your heart will never lie to you. There will be no mistakes, unless you resist your heart. If you choose to go against it, it will show up in many ways. It could lead to mis-communication, or a quarrel with a loved one. Or it might even show up as ill-health, depending on how long you've remained mis-aligned.

Lessons have a way of coming through when we are not aligned with our true beliefs; when we have not followed our heart or listened to our intuition. Our inner guidance is our compass for life, but it can only truly guide us if we are open and willing to explore what it has to offer. It's a two-way street. Honour your heart, trust your inner guidance and allow your intuition to guide you. Let the miracles flow, one by one.

You are enough, now

Are you playing the waiting game?

Many people wait...they may wait for the right time, when they have more money, when they are more qualified, feel more confident...etc.

The list could go on endlessly, if you let it.

But what if you didn't have to wait; how would that make you feel?

One of the most common reasons why people wait is because they feel they are not good enough. They start comparing themselves with others and this can bring up inadequacies they may not have even realised they had! How things trigger us can be a funny thing. One minute you might be casually going about your day and then, suddenly, you come across something on TV, or while scrolling through your social media feed – and you're suddenly riled up, for no particular reason. Or perhaps you see someone in an exotic location, or showing off their latest car – and suddenly your cheeks have heated up and your temper has begun to rise.

Does any of this sound familiar? Welcome, to the world of the green-eyed monster, which lays dormant in all of us until someone or something comes along that brings out the worst in us – *jealousy*. Suddenly the laid-back, pleasant human being you've always been doesn't seem so laid-back or nice, after all!

But, before you get caught up in slating your very existence, or wondering how you can possibly end up thinking this way, stop!

Remember, everything happens for a reason and that includes those little things that come up and provoke us. When they do, step back and take a deep breath in and then slowly exhale. Relax; you are only human and this is all part and parcel of being the awesome person that you are. Instead of burying this emotion, let's look at working 'with' it and allowing it to help us.

Let's uncover the real reason why this situation has got to you. More often than not, the real reason for becoming hot under the collar could be that the person you feel jealous towards is doing something that you tend to only dream about. Perhaps you think you should be in their shoes; you should have that new object – that lovely car or even their lovely lifestyle. You know what, though? You are right!

If you are able to travel, why shouldn't you be jetting off to an exotic destination? Why haven't you got that latest shiny object? And why aren't you living your dream life? How come that other person is doing it, but not you? I hesitate to state the obvious, but perhaps they are doing something that you aren't. And maybe – just maybe – they think of things differently and see themselves in a different way to how you see yourself. They probably see themselves in a positive light and – here's the thing – they feel they deserve those good things. Why? Because they realise they are worthy.

I know this 'truth bomb' may not be quite what you want to hear. And, while there's no magic pill that you can take to instantly change your life, you can look at it in a different way. After all, isn't it exciting to know that you can actually do something about this situation, *instead* of just 'dreaming' about it?

Let's start by building yourself up in such a way that you can see just how amazing you are. Remember, unless you can see it, others may not do so.

One way of overcoming any difficult pattern is to dig deeper. First off let's get to the bottom of why you were triggered by that situation where you felt jealous. Ask yourself, what's the real reason you want to wait? Journal this – and keep on asking yourself questions, until you get to the bottom of it.

If it helps you, go through all your great qualities and the things you can do that others can't. Perhaps, for example, you have a particular gift, you're amazing at organising or are really creative – etc.

Then ask yourself, 'How do I feel now?'

Are you feeling better? Great! Now take all this positive energy and ask yourself the following question, 'What is holding me back from going for what I want in life?'

I am guessing that the real answer is, 'Nothing!' Do you want to know why? Well, I have some good news for you.

It's because, you are good enough NOW.

Appreciate yourself

Take a moment to step back and survey all you have accomplished and the wonderful person that you are. Take a deep breath and really appreciate yourself. True appreciation comes from within. It gives meaning to life. It also gives a reason – to just be.

In a world filled with people trying to be like somebody else, be yourself!

I invite you to step fully into this moment of space and take time to soak in the ambience of appreciation for yourself.

Cheers to a more fulfilled you!

CHAPTER 6

Let love lead the way

Let love lead the way

Love goes a long way. It steers us through our lives, driving us through every stage of it. Let love lead the way through the next stage of your life. When love is at the core of everything you do, only good can happen. Let love be your foundation and build upon that with an open heart, filled with goodness and an abundance of gratitude. In moments of doubt, let love lead the way and light up your path. Let it be the blessing that carries your joy.

Be at one with love

Be at one with love. Place love at the heart of everything you do and all you stand for. Let it feed and replenish your soul with goodness. Enjoy the feeling it brings and allow joy to exude out of every pore and become your essence. Bask completely in these moments of bliss and let them engulf everything about you, for you *are* love.

Celebrate the unity and peace love gives and let it flow in abundance, as you touch others hearts with the true essence and spirit of what it means to give love, feel loved and be love.

Unity

When mind, body and spirit are connected, that is when you feel aligned and in balance. Everything just flows effortlessly and without resistance. This is because you are in harmony with yourself on the inside and it reflects on the outside, too. You produce an air of deep happiness from within, which radiates to others in wonderful ways.

Many activities can create this feeling. You could be sitting quietly by a stream, watching the world go by from a window, or while going for a leisurely stroll. Take a note of the things you do to help create this experience; this way, it can be repeated.

Enjoy the experience and really tap into the peace and joy it brings. You may find it useful to 'anchor' this feeling – for example, by squeezing your forefinger and thumb together. This sets a reminder in place, so that each time you want to feel balanced and connected you can simply squeeze your forefinger and thumb together again, which will trigger that same set of feelings.

This can be particularly helpful if you are feeling scattered and bewildered; those times when things are getting a little too much and you want a token of calm, in a messy space.

Being able to tap into this feeling of being at one with yourself, at will, can help in immeasurable ways. The ability to control and work with your mind, body and spirit offers creation of a deep connection with your soul. Building strength within the depths of your soul can lead to a happier and peaceful you. Surrender to the unity within, as you allow yourself to flourish and watch the magic happen.

Just because

When I was younger, I wouldn't do anything unless it had a purpose. For instance, I would only get up very early in order to exercise. I would walk somewhere only with a clear reason, or to reach a specific destination. I would write a song only to record it.

Now that I am older, I realise that nobody needs a reason to do something. You can do anything simply for the enjoyment of it; you may want to take a stroll just because you feel like it! You might sing because it brings you joy.

Keeping yourself open to the basic beauty of life can lead to immeasurable happiness. It allows you to tap into the spontaneity of life in its purest form; that, in itself, can be so much fun!

Flexibility gives you space to do the things you may not have been willing to try out, especially if you have a restrictive routine. If you can allow time for movement and growth, it can lead to expansion in many ways, including mentally, physically and on an energetic level.

Pause for a moment and think about a time that something beautiful happened when you least expected it. Such moments may seem crazy at the time, especially if you feel frustrated about not doing something you normally do. But they can lead to opportunities that you would not have contemplated, even in your wildest dreams.

Take inspired thoughts as an example. Nobody can wilfully make ideas happen; they just appear like magic, out of the blue and often after you have been doing something completely different – like watching a movie or going out for the day. You can't control this; the ideas just happen. When they do, it is wise not to disrupt the flow. Instead, just go with it – let it be.

Nature, is beautiful to watch. It is easy to get absorbed into the magic of it all. Everything is so exquisitely orchestrated. Bees fly around, collecting pollen from flowers that sway in perfect unison in the breeze; birds chirp in a reassuring way, almost as if to say "Everything is going to be all right". It all works like clockwork; each plays a part in a beautifully designed tapestry of wildlife, completely unaided by us. We have only to admire nature's masterpiece, as we gaze upon its glory in majestic awe.

Try flowing through your day, now and then, noticing the feeling this brings. You will likely find yourself feeling lighter and softer, rather like a ballerina, effortlessly sliding across the floor – or a beautiful swan, gliding across a lake in blissful harmony. This offers calm and contentment, with the sense that you are completely at ease, reassured that all is well in your world. As you're more likely to then greet others with a ready smile, they, too, can benefit from this gentle, soft energy you are giving out.

Everything merges into one, as we are all connected in love and light, like magnetic waves drifting in and out of each other's lives.

Surrender to this feeling of 'just because', every now and then; it can take you further than you ever imagined and make you happier than you thought possible. Just like with a child playing 'make believe', create your own sense of play – just because.

Calm

Give yourself the gift of peace and quiet. Be at peace with yourself and with those around you. Being at peace is part of being whole and complete. No words are needed and no expression is required.

Time

Just be in the moment and allow yourself to accept the most generous gift there is; the gift of time. Time cannot be taken back or withheld. Give it graciously to those you care about. Allow yourselves to enjoy time together as well as having time to yourself. Being in the moment and only focusing on what is at hand – and who you are with – can bring some of the most rewarding feelings. Use your time wisely and consciously.

Rhythm of life

Having a routine is like getting into a rhythm of life. It helps us to create boundaries and maintain structure. It's a method of building blocks, one piece at a time that helps us to stand tall. Supported by this solid foundation, we stay strong and are fully equipped, ready for all that life has in store for us.

Sometimes you have to disconnect, in order to reconnect with yourself and your loved ones.

Remember to Pause

In times of uncertainty and doubt, take time to pause. It allows you time to think and decide what's right for you. It gives you much-needed space. It helps to release pressure in times of stress and brings relief to the most chaotic of situations. A pause can make the difference between what's right or wrong. While many people may urge you to hurry, remember to pause.

Wellbeing

A little bit of most things is better than a whole lot of one thing or not enough of the other. There's a time to work, a time to eat, a time to sleep and a time to have fun. Making space for these, in proportion, will help you maintain a balanced life. A more balanced life leads to a happier and more fulfilled you. It is this general understanding – and knowing that all is well in your world – that makes it possible for you to have an overall better sense of wellbeing. If we can find a way to be at one with one another and let love lead the way, we hold the potential to bring more peace into our lives.

CHAPTER 7

Be happy now

Be happy now

There is a common misconception that happiness lies in the future and is something to be striven for. It is almost as though you have to wait to be happy. What is it that you are waiting for, exactly? Some people think they have to 'have more' or 'be more', to achieve happiness. For instance, they'll be happy when they receive a million pounds, or when they win the lottery, when they become thinner or when they retire. What if you could be happy now, just by being the way you are and looking exactly as you do? How would that make you feel? Fabulous, I expect!

Happiness begins from within

Happiness is often thought of as an end goal, but looking at it this way could keep you limited to thinking that you're unable to be happy now. Instead, try thinking of happiness as a journey, not a destination. You don't need an event to take place, or require permission from others to achieve this.

Happiness begins from within.

Repeat that again, out loud. Happiness begins from within – and it begins with you. This can be quite profound, once you get your head around it.

Decide to be happy

Give yourself permission to be happy. It's a choice. Say to yourself, "I choose happiness"; set it as your intention. The moment you decide to be happy (yes, I said 'decide', because everything stems from making a decision) that is when you can start feeling that way, unashamedly.

There may be times when things happen around us that can affect our behaviour, of course. It is up to us to choose how to respond and react to the situations, events and other people around us. It is up to you to take responsibility for your own state of mind, which includes being happy. Notice I said 'being'; we are happiest when we allow ourselves to just 'be', which means being and staying present in the moment. While it's nice to reminisce about times gone by – and the happiness we experienced previously – it is even more rewarding to start making new memories now, experiencing joy today.

Happiness tools

It's not always easy to be happy, I know. But you can help yourself by doing some things to help place you in the happy zone faster. For instance, I often find playing music loudly and dancing around the room cheers me up immensely. Music is like magic; it can transport you to another dimension, instantly, serving as the perfect, quick pick-me-up. Dancing is movement, which can also help lift your spirits. It's a form of exercise, too, which is terrific for grounding and taking you out of your head, away from what's troubling you. Serotonin and 'feel-good' hormones, release while you move, enabling you to start feeling brighter, offering a much more positive outlook on life.

If you're at work, or somewhere that you can't do much in the way of physical activity, a quick spritz of a favourite scent or perfume can work wonders for your morale, giving an instant boost. As you inhale the perfume, it's as though a sudden burst of excitement has hit your senses. A combination of the touch, as the scent kisses your skin, and its distinct aroma, can be a sudden reminder of how wonderful you are and how great your life is.

Keep smiling

I recall a time when I was working for a well-known bank. I was smiling, at the time. I was fairly new to the place and it was a very quiet and serious atmosphere; hardly anyone talked to one another. My manager, noticing I had a smile on my face, said to me, "You're smiling. Well, we'll soon find a way to wipe that off your face." I was taken aback, although that actually made me smile even more – my rebellious streak coming out, I guess. I discovered, later, that he had an unusual sense of humour. I didn't let his attitude change me, however. I kept on smiling anyway, regardless of the work culture in that place.

Smiling can brighten up even the darkest of days! When you smile at someone it can lift their mood, too. Even though you may not feel like it, try making an effort to smile more often; it will make a difference to your outlook on life.

Another way of reminding yourself of how wonderful you are is to regularly say things that you love about yourself. You can say them in front of a mirror – perhaps first thing in the morning. Try this out and notice how good it makes you feel. If you are apprehensive about doing this so, take it slowly; start by focusing on one good thing at a time. If it helps, write it down beforehand. Smiling at yourself in the mirror is always a good place to start.

Kindness is key

Kindness is key to leading a happy life. While it's easier to be kind to others, it isn't always easy to be gentle on ourselves. Especially in the case of women, we can tend to put others needs before ourselves. But, remember, we have a duty to care for ourselves, too. You are vital to your circle of life. If it wasn't for you, there are so many things that wouldn't happen or run smoothly. As I've mentioned before, you matter. Please remember to be kind to yourself, too, whether this means taking time out to do the things you love, or taking things at a slower pace. Nurturing your mind, body and soul will really help your wellbeing – and this is all part of you being happy.

Now and again, it's good to take a step back and look at the bigger picture. Rather than just working constantly and rushing around, often moving on to the next project swiftly after finishing the previous task. Take the time to really appreciate all that you are. This can include things that you have achieved as well as just appreciating you for being you.

Celebrations don't only belong to others. You have a right to shout out and celebrate your successes, too. By doing so, you will likely attract more opportunities for success. As they say, 'like attracts like', so be proud of your accomplishments, however large or small. May your happiness be evident to many and any tears shed be few.

Let laughter be your signature and love be your mantra.

Make it your mission to be happy

You don't have to justify being happy. There are no rules. No one has a right to stop you being happy. Nobody can keep you from being happy unless you allow them to. Don't give others power over your state of mind. Don't allow their opinions or attitudes to dim your beautiful, inner sparkle. Happiness is a matter of choice and it's up to you take the step to make it.

Cups full of happiness

Do things that bring you joy and fill you with happiness. When you feel good, you attract more love and light into your world. This is then reflected in how you are, with others around you. A simple smile can make all the difference in brightening someone's day. Pour your cups full of happiness on to everyone you meet. Nourish your soul with kindness and speak to others the way you'd like to be spoken to. Add a little humour to the mix and you've got yourself a recipe for happiness!

Happiness works wonders for the soul.

Remember, you deserve to be happy, so be happy now.

CHAPTER 8

Resilience

Ups and downs

Life involves many ups and downs. Sometimes the downs can occur when we least expect them, involving quite a shock. I recall when I had a gardening accident and it caused limited use of my right hand. As that's my dominant hand, it completely knocked me back. I felt that my world had fallen apart. I found I couldn't do the most basic of things by myself; things like bathing, brushing my hair, making a drink, or cooking. I had to rely on others for many things. On top of it all, I had to give up working at a school, which I had loved doing. What had started out as a good intention (i.e. getting the garden done) ended up with my world being turned upside down.

Step by step

This incident taught me so much about other people, however, and a great deal about myself. It was such a tough time, involving impatience, alongside anger and tears of frustration, but I learnt so much from it. I learnt to be strong, patient, understanding and resilient. At first, I felt that I couldn't move forward from the initial incident. But, gradually, step by step, taking a day at a time I managed to place one foot in front of the other. Through that I gained an ability to see further than my immediate circumstance. What had appeared as a bleak and unfortunate situation was actually a pivotal moment in my life. If this incident hadn't happened I might not even be writing this book today!

I know it's said that everything happens for a reason, and sometimes that sounds so clichéd. Yet, I now believe that everything does have a place and a purpose – even if it doesn't feel like it at the time.

Trust

I had to tap into resources that I never realised I had! It didn't happen overnight, like a lightning bolt; it took time and perseverance. I also had to put a tremendous amount of energy and discipline into to it, because I was determined to change the situation – not just for myself, but for my family, as well. I remember wondering what kind of example I would be setting my son, if I just gave up. No – that wasn't an option at all. I didn't know how and I didn't know when, but I knew that things would improve, because they had to. I had a deep sense of knowing that this wasn't how things were meant to be. Perhaps you're familiar with that kind of knowing. It might occur when you wake in the middle of the night – knowing that what you're seeing isn't aligned with your desire for greatness. Such feelings can be quite profound.

This can be when you most need to trust your feelings and step into them more. Call upon everything you have, and let inspired action guide you through to another level. No one has all the answers and sometimes you just have to follow your instinct, letting it carry you to the next stage. There are no rules and you can ignore those who judge you. This process takes as long as it takes but, often, before you know it, you can get back on track – or at a place that is even greater than before.

Inner work

I used visualisation techniques, when I was recovering from injury, to picture myself being able to do the things I loved again. This included playing musical instruments, as well as working out without the need to hold on to something – as my balance was affected. I did some very painful exercises, regularly, to help regain movement in my hand. The doctors didn't think surgery would be any use, so I had to try other methods to improve my condition. I also did inner work, refusing to give up and give in. I regularly said affirmations out loud, like 'I am getting better and better with every moment'. I prayed and listened for answers, which were then given to me by divine inspiration. One of these was to bathe my hand in warm water, alongside massaging it – and, of course, resting it. The doctor told me to take painkillers whenever it hurt. I did so to begin with and then practised energy healing; I imagined a white light healing my hand and, at night, pictured regeneration taking place while I slept.

While all this was taking place, I also followed my intuition to start a business. This came about after I had received a compliment in the surgery waiting room, before my physiotherapy appointment. 'SommerSparkle' was soon born – an online jewellery and accessories business, bringing beautiful jewellery to those who want to look amazing and feel fabulous. I knew I had the intention of wanting to spread love and help make women feel special – and supplied pieces particularly suited to those preparing for a special occasion. My entrepreneurial journey had begun! The business has since gone on to win multiple awards, internationally and still thrives today. If it hadn't been for the injury I endured, none of this may have happened!

I now see setbacks as opportunities for greatness, in disguise. Yes, they are devastating at the time, but there's always the greater picture. Just like an artist can never truly appreciate the finished painting, until he or she steps back after it has been completed, you will never fully understand the lesson in this part of your story until it has been told.

You are mighty

Think back to low times in your past – we all have them – and notice how much stronger you are now, because of them. If you could overcome them before, you can do so again. It doesn't have to be the end of the world, when a low patch occurs; many times, it can be the beginning of a brand new chapter in your life. So, get back up, raise your head and recognise your beauty and strength. You are stronger than you ever imagined! Take these moments and make them matter; gaze upon them like stepping stones, to a stronger and more resilient you.

You have so got this. You are mighty!

CHAPTER 9

You are a survivor

Running away

There have been a few times in my life when all I wanted to do was run away. Indeed, a couple of times I did just that, in an effort to escape from my current situation – and perhaps even to start afresh completely. These episodes still haunt me now. It's an awful feeling to be cornered, with no place else to go, and nobody to turn to. In this situation it can be like being a caged tiger lashing out at the nearest thing to it, or doing what is least expected. In that type of situation, running away seemed like the only option open to me – and a good idea, at the time.

Speaking up

Being an introvert, I tend to shy away from confrontation until I'm particularly passionate about something. If I see an injustice being done, especially, people then see a different side to me – an erupting, volcanic side, which is far from pleasant but certainly gets the message across. Like the time I saw a child being bullied on a bus by an elderly lady, who riled up the other people next to her to 'side' with her against the child (who was just getting on the bus). I spotted the unfairness of a child being shouted at, just because they didn't realise something about their bus pass. I saw that they were alone, without anyone to stick up for them, so I stepped forward, boldly and told the 'others' that they should know better, because their behaviour was far from fair. They soon stopped yelling! Another lady on the bus thanked me for sticking up for that child while no one else would. Many people have a tendency to stand with the majority, or with those that shout the loudest. When you are passionate about something, or defending somebody else, it's often easier to speak up. But it isn't always so easy to stand up and speak up when the person who is being victimised is you.

Things have to change

I know countless women – and, indeed, a couple of men – who have been in abusive relationships. Whether involving physical or mental abuse, there are some things they all have in common. They may try to play down the situation, at first, in an effort to trick themselves into believing everything is okay. They then think they're responsible for provoking the other person and, if only they could behave a certain way – not answer back, or be more submissive – their abuser would suddenly start treating them better. This is seldom the case, however. I recall one incident – a very serious one - where a woman told me about a turning-point event that made her realise she had to take drastic action – and fast. Prepare yourself for this, as it is quite a shocking incident. It relates to when her husband held her over the balcony of a high storey flat; in that precarious, terrifying and life-threatening situation, he made her promise that, from then on, she would do as he said. It was only when she literally saw her life flash before her eyes, that she knew things had to change. So she gradually built up some money, whilst also gathering up the courage to leave him. When she told me about this, I was horrified – as, indeed, you may have been, in reading the same. It sent a chill right through to my bones. I couldn't believe somebody could do this to another human being, especially to someone they apparently loved! To make things worse, this guy seemed really down-to-earth and friendly, in everyday life.

The lady in this situation was very well esteemed and high up in her industry; she seemed a bold, go-getter. Nobody would have guessed that these things were going on for her, behind closed doors.

Starting again

After the lady in question left her husband, she had to get an injunction out against him. She eventually filed for divorce. Fortunately, they didn't have any children together, so no other contact was made. She built herself up again. She read self-help books, had therapy, and worked on her self-esteem and qualities. She had to start all over again. In doing so, she put loving herself at the top of her agenda. She essentially had to rebuild herself to a version that was much more resilient than before. I'm relieved and delighted to say that she is now happily remarried, with two adorable children – and what happened before seems like a distant memory. She is so far removed from the person she was before, that it almost seems like her past happened to someone else she once knew – or even to a stranger.

For people who are going through a rough situation, no matter how bleak it seems, remember that 'everything is temporary'. It's a theme I featured in a previous book: *Life Lessons from a 40 something…: For The Best Start In Life*. Things can change for the better if you want them to. It all starts with you. You call the shots in your life. There is light at the end of the tunnel!

Phoenix rising

If you have gone through a similar situation – perhaps you are separated, divorced or your kids have flown the nest – remember, you are not alone. Be gentle and take things one day at a time, one step at a time. No one can tell you how to think or feel, and you can go at your own pace. You need to fall in love with you again and rebuild yourself, inside and out. Start with doing what you love: read self-help and self-love books if you like reading; go out for walks in the forest; take up that hobby again that you always enjoyed.

Remember, you had a life before any of those relationships and can do so again. Your light will begin to shine again. It starts with a flicker. You can do this, Beautiful!

Reaching out

Life has many ups and downs; it's not always plain sailing. The turbulent moments can, however, also help us appreciate the calmer, quieter moments. When unwanted and dramatic things happen, it's easy to feel isolated. You may feel like you're the only one going through this and that nobody cares or understands. Empty and alone are two of the most debilitating feelings a person can feel. At times like those, it can seem that you have nowhere to turn; whether physically or mentally. You can feel almost paralysed from taking any action. It might be hard enough to think straight, let alone take any physical form of action.

Under such conditions, your judgement can appear misguided, causing the lines between friend and foe to become blurred. Frightened yet defensive; cold and in pain. You may be hurting and full of sorrow for yourself. You may even worry that you're a disappointment to those around you – including those who you thought you could trust and vice versa. I know this feeling because I have felt this type of pain, deep down to my core – lost and afraid and all too eager to feel loved. Sometimes, the deeper you fall, the more you feel, even though you don't want to have more depth of feeling! At the same time, you may have a sense of numbness that no words can explain; it's like all hope has gone. At that point in time, you can't think of anything to smile about—not a single thing!

That's when it's time to reach out to someone, and it doesn't matter who. Whether you reach out to a professional or a friend, it's by talking that you'll begin to see things in a new light.

This will help put you on the road to a happier you.

Step into your 'brave'

Take heart, for this is the moment that you can truly get in touch with your inner warrior and tap into resources that seem to exist from a time gone by. You may feel an almost familiar sense of bravery. You can almost taste, touch and hear familiar sounds that have long been forgotten. Search inside your soul — it's there! Look again; there it is!

That's it – you've been here before. Memories now start flooding back to you. Your heart may begin to beat a little faster and perhaps your pulse starts to race. Think back to a time when you needed this feeling and when you felt this courage; a time when what you had to do took over in a way that was actually more important than what you were feeling inside.

The queen within you

Look up and rise up! Recognise the queen within you. Feel her; the one with passion, determination and nerves of steel. The one with an inner strength that can fight harder than a raging bull, if the need arises. Search your soul, sister and take charge of your life. Take control and take back your power. Search your deepest senses and let nothing stand in your way. There is more to you than meets the eye. You will not be defeated by these seemingly bleak times, because deep inside you is a defiant nature, with a will to overcome and succeed. You'll get through this; you always have done and always will. While there's blood in your veins and passion in your heart, you won't stop, because you are a survivor!

Decisions can be empowering. Everything starts with a decision, whether good or bad.

You have two options: you can either go with the wind or you can thrive. Which will you choose?

CHAPTER 10

Empower yourself

Stay true to you

We grow up looking for approval from others. It's only natural to want to please our parents and caregivers, as a child – but, as an adult, things are somewhat different.

As you discover your own identity and celebrate your individuality, realise that it's not always wise to do as others do – or even to think like others. You'll eventually discover more about yourself, about your own, hidden depths and why you do things a certain way. You'll realise that you differ from others and that it's okay to be yourself – even if others don't agree.

Betrayal

Have you ever felt betrayed by the person you cared about the most – and whom you thought felt the same way? If you have; you probably felt very angry. You could even stay angry forever, but that wouldn't help you in the long run. Why not use the anger to fuel your vision, instead?

It's time to gather up your courage and work with the enemy within that's keeping negative feelings buried inside you. Try bringing them to the surface and releasing them. Only then will you have the power to move on and take control of your feelings. You are better than this and are worth far much more.

Hold your ground, as you stand in grace and dignity and watch the magic unfold into something beautiful.

Sometimes it can be tough, especially if it feels like the whole world is at odds with you – and that not a single soul understands where you're coming from. At times like these, you may consider giving in and just going along with what others think and feel – anything for a quiet life. But this is the easy way out. That may not seem obvious, at first. But, deep down inside, you know the feeling when something is not quite right. It might be an uneasy feeling you get at the base of your stomach – and you just know something has to change. Perhaps you know that you're betraying your soul, in favour of others.

Don't give your power away to others, Beautiful! It's time to roll up your sleeves and step into your power zone.

I know it may seem hard, but this is the time when you can't just let it be. Things have a way of coming out and sometimes at the most inopportune and unexpected moments. I think you'll understand what I mean.

Inner strength

This is when you need to search deep inside. Take time to not only think, but to also feel deeply; know what it is that you are yearning for. Close your eyes, if it helps. Reach within your heart and soul, allowing yourself to tap into your inner power. Remember, your inner strength has always been there and will never leave you – even if you have betrayed yourself at some point.

Feel the energy vibrate from deep within you; grab it, hold on to it and let it pour out of you, like lava filling up a volcano that's erupting in all its glory. Now you have summoned up the courage you need, to be the person you are truly meant to be.

Stand tall and embrace your inner glory. Notice how others look in amazement, as you reveal your true colours – ones that you've kept hidden for many years.

Now that you've discovered what you are made of, feel brave in the knowledge that you, alone, hold the key to this. You alone have the power to tap into your inner strength at any given moment, whenever you need it. There's no need to be afraid any longer. You had it all along; it was just inside you, waiting for the right moment to come out. Now, go and take charge of your life and beam in the brightness of your inner strength!

What serves you

You have the right to have standards; it doesn't make you odd, selfish or snobbish. If someone asks you to take part in something, or to go somewhere you just don't feel right with, then don't go along with it just to try to fit in. Like a square peg in a round hole, if it doesn't feel right to you now, it also won't feel right then. Learn to value your opinions and stay true to what serves you. Other people may not fully understand, but you will be respected in the long run.

Say 'no'

Don't be afraid of saying 'no', once in a while. It may seem unnatural; it might not even be in your regular vocabulary, but you'll be amazed at how much better you feel after you've got used to saying it. It will also help free up time for you to focus on the things and people who mean a lot to you. This approach will eliminate confusion and give you gumption. Don't be a follower; be a leader of your own life.

Do what feels right

Always stay true to what you believe in and go with what feels right. Doing the opposite won't help you in the long run and may also confuse the people around you. Trust yourself and stay tuned to your inner compass. This will guide you to many great things in life and steer you towards what makes you happy.

Empower yourself

Don't wait for others to 'big you up', to acknowledge and support you; you could be waiting forever! Practise going within and encouraging yourself. Be your own cheerleader and value yourself; your opinions, feelings and what you contribute to life all matter. *You* matter. Encourage, motivate and find it within you to empower yourself. Do so in such a way that there are no doubts in your mind as to where you are coming from. Be relentless in your pursuit to achieve all you want out of life.

Use your inner power to fill you with grace and positivity. Dress like you mean it, walk like you own it, and live like there's no tomorrow. Be the person you have always wanted to be, with a sprinkle of style and pizazz thrown in for good measure.

Celebrate you

Celebrate yourself, flawless in the knowledge that only you know how very hard you've worked to get here. Only you know how you've wept and wiped away so many tears, perhaps while hearing laughter from others. Only you know the pain you have overcome to get where you are now. So, make sure you celebrate with all your heart, your soul and your mind. Nobody deserves this more than you do. So, go celebrate, Lovely! No one can rock this like you can.

CHAPTER 11

Master reframing

Master reframing

Experience brings with it great gifts. There are many highs – and a few lows thrown in, just to keep you on your toes. They don't even have to be bad experiences, even though they may feel that way at the time. It will depend on how you view things. Perspective can turn what you first thought was the 'end of the world' into a learning curve of sorts. This can then be thought of as a gift; a chance for you to gain strength and grow from the experience.

One of the tools that has helped me, immensely, is learning how to reframe things. It takes a little practice, but, once you've grasped the general idea, you'll soon get the hang of it. I now do this without even realising it; so much so, that someone recently nicknamed me a 'master of reframing'!

How to reframe

If you're not familiar with this technique, the following exercise will help. It's particularly useful for when feeling upset:

- Write down your problem or situation

- Now write down your thoughts about the problem

- Express your feelings on the paper, writing down how you feel – and perhaps why you feel like this

- Now, explore a few different ways of looking at the matter, especially ways that are more positive and beneficial to you

- Read these fresh ideas over to yourself

- Write down your thoughts after reading this new perspective

- Now, write down your feelings and emotions with this fresh outlook in mind

- How do you feel now?

Be patient with yourself when you first try this exercise, as it can take a little practice before you become used to doing it. Soon, you'll be reframing automatically and may not even need to write it down, but write it down until you get used to it. It sometimes helps, seeing things written down. Another thing that can help is if you start looking for evidence to support your positive statement. This reinforces what you're saying and serves as confirmation, to yourself, that you're on the right track. This extra step may not always be necessary. Just feeling better could be confirmation enough.

Package it up

Reframing is to do with how you package up and position things in your mind, so that you're able to move forward in a way that supports and empowers you. It lets you change something bad into something good, and can be a positive turning point. You may already be doing it, without even realising. It's a little like seeing the good in every situation, focusing on the benefits. This transformation can be incredible!

Reframing examples

In my earlier days, when I was growing up, my mother's response to the plans I had for my band was that I was 'building castles in the sky'. Although I was upset at her remark, at the time, in later years I saw it in another way. A fresh perspective allowed me to position it to myself differently, which was far more positive and uplifting. By giving it new meaning – changing it from being something often thought of as a negative phrase – it transformed into a positive and powerful statement. So much so, that it became the inspiration for my second book, '*Building Castles In The Sky: How To Make Your Dreams Come True*'.

What happened for me, internally, in that reframing, was that I agreed with her, in saying, 'Yes, I *am* building castles in the sky,' but continued the train of thought with, 'you have to be able to build castles in the sky first, before they are made into something concrete and 'built' on land.' In other words, I was thinking that you have to have the idea in your head first, before you turn them into reality. The thought almost always precedes the action and then materialises into something you can see and touch.

Looking back, I am so glad that we had that conversation then, otherwise I may never have written that book and been able to help others along the way! For me, it reinforced that notion that everything happens for a reason.

Another story of reframing is a time when a lady smiled at me and, glaring down at my stomach, said, 'You look so well'. I just smiled and took it as a well-intentioned compliment and said, 'Thank you. I feel much healthier'. I knew she was implying that I'd gained a few pounds since she had last seen me, but I quickly changed the meaning around in my head. I chose to take her comment at face value and was pleasant to her in my response.

Those are just a couple of stories about reframing; I expect you can think of many more.

Make it work for you

Some people can't help themselves in their habit of expressing their thoughts and feelings naturally and openly, regardless of hurting yours. I can almost guarantee that there will be many chances, therefore, for you to practice the art of reframing!

Remember the reason why you are mastering this technique. It's not an excuse to lash back at someone being rude or be impolite. It's intended to make their comment work for you, in a way that supports you. Then you can move forward in a positive, loving and caring way that should feel more empowering. This is a tool. Make it work for you and you'll be a reframing queen in no time!

The next time someone says something unkind or unsupportive, reposition it to yourself in a positive way. Flip the script! Put this in the power bank of tools you are building up, because you never know when it'll come in handy.

This can be used to transform anything bad into something good; to change a negative into a positive, or to move a 'No way' into a 'Why not?'. Watch those frowns turn upside down! You'll be a reframing ninja in next to no time, as you create the habit of seeing solutions, instead of problems. This will help you step out of the shadows and live your life in a more positive light.

CHAPTER 12

It's absolutely never too late

The gift of experience

You have so much to offer. You can still walk into a room and turn heads (if that's what you want). Life doesn't have to pass you by, unless you let it. Do that thing you have always wanted to do. Work on a plan to visit that place you've always wanted to go to. Prepare for that adventure, in a way that you know it's going to happen.

You have got the gift of experience behind you, which is an invaluable asset and something to be proud of. And most of all, you get to be a better version of your former self because you have more to bring to the table. Play brighter. This is a wonderful time to be you! Remember, you don't need anybody else's approval to go after what you want in life.

A truer version of yourself

Moving on to a new stage in your life is all about evolving, adapting and being your best self. This takes effort and courage and may not always be easy, as you meet challenges along the way. But overcoming these shows strength and the process means you'll acquire skills and achieve things that you never dreamt possible, before. You will become more of who you are meant to be. It's not about getting older; it's about becoming a better and truer version of yourself. You may be tough and dynamic, at times; kind and loving at others. As women, we tend to have a hard, 'Don't-mess-with-me' side, chiselled with a gentler, softer and more refined side. Both are equally important and help make up who we are.

Don't fall into the trap of thinking you're too old to be or do something; more often than not this just isn't the case. Although occasionally it will be true, for instance, if you want to be a fashion model or sports person, where you need to appear a certain way, or be at a particular fitness level. But most of the

114

time you can do what you have always
wanted to. Think of age as another number
and a magnificent milestone you have
accomplished.

Be the queen of your kingdom

You deserve to be happy; you are still worthy.
There is no need to place yourself as a mere
observer of life. If you feel the urge go ahead
and take centre stage, you have just as much
right to go and do that. Be the star of the
show and the queen of your kingdom!

Be vivacious

Be vivacious and carefree in your actions, and
radiate exuberance. It's okay to show that you
are happy, too. We can often play down being
happy, for fear that it'll be frowned upon by
others. We may feel we are 'showing off' in
front of others. For many people, this stems
from childhood, especially if they were told
off for it. Perhaps you were told that, as a girl,
you should be more reserved. But, as we get
older, the same 'rules' no longer apply. You
don't need an excuse to be happy. Wanting
this is an innate desire – I would even go so

far as to say it's a basic, human need. I know a couple of women who almost feel guilty for feeling happy, at any point, as though it's a guilty pleasure. Happiness is not just for men, or young teenagers without responsibility. It's for everyone. It is never too late to start doing things that make you happy. Start now – and watch how it changes you.

Been there, done that

If you start doing something and discover that it's not for you, after all, then simply stop doing it – or change it for another activity. You don't have to stay at it, until you have completed so many weeks, years, etc. If you're not enjoying it, or it doesn't serve you, then stop! The likelihood is, you're at that stage in life where you've 'Been there, done that' and don't need to waste time doing anything you really dislike. Life is too short for that. If you feel guilty about letting someone else down, perhaps because it's something you did together and they still want to pursue it, just explain that it's not for you and let them continue. The chances are, they'll completely understand. They may even be a little relieved; perhaps they had already picked up, from your behaviour, that you weren't as into the same activity as they were. It's always easier and more enjoyable when both participants are enthusiastic about the same thing.

Who are you really living your life for?

If you have a habit of worrying about what other people think, then ask yourself who it is you're really living your life for. If you're living your life for you, it doesn't matter what other people think about your plans and chosen activities. Nobody has a right to dictate what you can or can't do. They haven't walked in your shoes or felt things the way you have – just as you haven't with theirs. If the person is a sibling, or your son or daughter, then sit down and explain to them why you want to do something – and reiterate how it makes you feel. Remember that they probably feel they are protecting you and looking after you. It will be out of their love for you that they react as they do. Once they see the glint in your eyes, however – spotting your enthusiasm, and the excitement your

117

choice brings you – they'll have a better understanding. Then they're likely to show less resistance.

Look ahead

It can be lovely to look back at old times, when you were younger and full of excitement and wondered at what lay ahead at the world in front of you. However, doing this too often can stunt your growth, inhibiting your potential in the present.

Yes, reminiscing can feel terrific and may even help to re-ignite passion within you. It may give you the energy and the optimism to follow a pursuit or dream you once had, but, for one reason or another, didn't fully happen. There is, however, also another possible side to this: regrets.

Regrets can have you crying over misspent younger days, especially where you miss something that is no more. You may feel empty about your present situation or, even worse, hopeless about the future.

Some people strive to look younger in the hope that in some way, they will also *feel* younger – perhaps more alive.

Another element of this is where people just want to be loved and – above all – feel loved. They are often mis-led into thinking that it's only the young who are truly loved, admired and appreciated. This is, of course, far from true.

Regrets are pointless because, no matter how hard you try, you can never return and change the past. Don't beat yourself up by saying, 'If only I could do it over again…', or 'If only I hadn't…'. Life has no time for 'if only'. Instead, focus on what you *can* do. Learn from your experiences and use this wealth of wisdom to help make better decisions and improve your existing circumstances.

You may have heard a similar expression to, 'Don't look behind you; you're not going in that direction'. That statement is true, to a certain extent. Stay present and enjoy the moment. Appreciate what you have now. You've got a lot more going for you than you realise. Once you've really drunk in all the joy you have, look ahead to the future and all the good things that lie ahead. If you're finding it hard to imagine these, start to make new plans for your future. They don't to be concrete but, sometimes, just having an idea can help you feel optimistic about life – and the many wonders it can bring.

Allow yourself to live in a world full of possibilities. The future is as bright as you want it to be. Make it bold, make it bright and, above all, make it yours. Remember, it's you who holds the keys to a happy life. You get to choose! It all begins with you, so, what are you going to do? Are you going to keep picturing what once was, wishing you were back there where you can't go, or will you look ahead to a brand new day and start getting excited about your life?

Don't be afraid at what the future holds. Embrace the excitement as you enjoy new adventures, make new discoveries and explore new experiences. Don't keep your dreams in your head; allow them to reveal themselves in your waking life, too, as you make way for the many opportunities that can unfold before you.

Keep moving forward and reach for those stars. It's absolutely never too late to follow your heart, your passion and your dreams.

CHAPTER 13

Reinvent yourself

Start over

There may be times when all you want to do is stay under the duvet and hide until the world has gone away. Maybe you're wishing you could disappear into a black hole over something that went wrong, thinking it's the end of the world. Think again!

This could be the perfect time for you to start over. Not in a destructive, 'I'm running away and never coming back' kind of way, but in an 'I'm introducing you to a brand new me' kind of way.

This is when reinvention steps in. It may seem a little daunting and perhaps even somewhat surprising. But, in all likelihood, there's an element of you that feels a little excited by the prospect. Go on, admit it!

Adventure— that's where it's at! The great thing is, you don't need anyone else to be on board with it. This is your journey; how you want to play the entire story is up to you. You decide. It's your ride. You get to choose how fast or slow you want to take it.

Reinvent yourself

If you don't like how you look, then change it. Reinvent yourself. It worked for icons like Madonna and David Bowie! Reinvention is the birth place of creativity. Have fun with it. Whether you feel the urge to cut your hair, or dramatically change its colour. Or you want to wear clothes that make you feel sexy and glamorous—just do it! It will dramatically recharge your life, giving you a much-needed boost. If you feel the desire to take up dance classes, or take part in amateur dramatics, just go ahead and book those classes – or find a group in your area to join. It doesn't matter how old you are. There are no age restrictions to having fun! If anything, increasing age is more of a reason to enjoy your life.

Transform your look

Start by looking at yourself in the mirror. How do you think you look? Could you have a bigger smile on your face? If the answer is 'Yes', then ask yourself what it is you actually want to change. Chances are, you really do love the way you look, but are too shy of admitting it in front of others. It's okay to be happy with your looks. Accentuate your best features and give them the attention they deserve. There is too much pressure, by far, placed on women to look for things to find fault in, in this regard. How about bigging yourself up now and again! It's a whole new ball game and builds up your self-esteem, in the process.

If you want a new hair-do, get it done; new clothes? Sort them! Do the things you've always wanted to; there's no need to ask the opinions of others around you. Besides, you already know you're gorgeous, don't you?

Transform your look in a way that makes you want to strut your stuff, in your own, feminine way.

What's in a name?

Are you happy with your name? More and more people are choosing to change their names. They're looking for something they prefer and identify better with. Nobody would have done this, a long time ago, for fear of being frowned upon – but in today's world it's okay. Even some celebrities have two identities. One is more like their real name and the other is a persona they create. Yes, it can be perceived to be divaesque, but does it really matter? If it makes you happy, then go with it.

There's a lot to be said about a name. One person may feel more flamboyant with one name, whilst someone else is more confident with another. It could be that you have always wished you could get up on stage to sing or speak but, as 'Anna', for example, you didn't feel you could to. Identifying with 'Candice', however, you suddenly feel you can do anything, and so are happy to jump on stage without a moment's hesitation. Sure, you may dress differently and even hold yourself in a different way. But, because you've created a whole new version of you, you have turned things around – and, in being 'Candice', you now feel more confident. Whatever the reason, if it makes you more like the person you want to be, then why not?

Personality

You don't have to officially change your name, of course, unless you want to. You could just take on the personality of your new character and use it to help you become the person you've always wanted to. Are you happy with your personality? Or would you rather be bolder and outspoken, or even quieter and calmer. Believe it or not, this too can be changed. It all starts with you deciding to be who you are. While you have your own individual traits, what's on the surface and how you appear to others can be altered – if only in small ways. It's a little like acting. Immerse yourself in that character and practice becoming the person you want to be. Rather than being inauthentic, this can actually enhance your original characteristics in a way that makes you more of who you are.

Getting into character – so to speak – can help you in many more ways, including exploring a new and more exciting - part of yourself. It's still you; just a brighter version of your true nature, coming out to play.

Go to that party

Dress up and go to that party! Put on that dazzling dress and wear your hair how you want to. I recall, when I was in my mid-thirties, how a hairdresser said that now I'm at a certain age I should have my hair short because it's more suitable for women of my age to do so. I was gobsmacked; I couldn't believe such audacity! Needless to say, I never went to that hairdresser again. It's the same with clothes. How you dress is up to you. As long as it suits you – and the image you want to portray – it really has little to do with others. That is, unless there's a necessary dress code, of course.

You are never too old to party or go clubbing to dance the night away. I remember, again, in my thirties, when I wanted to go dancing and my friends decided they were too old to go to clubs. I was astounded; I couldn't understand why they'd think that way. I obviously thought differently! You are never too old to dance. So, go to that party, sing along to that song, dance to your own heartbeat – and laugh to your heart's content.

Reinvention

Make life work for you, not the other way around. If you don't like your current circumstances, change them. If you dislike your weaknesses, then play to your strengths. See reinvention as a chance to create new opportunities and make a happier you. Be reborn as a lover of life and a creator of happiness.

CHAPTER 14

Glamour

Get glammed up!

Do you ever look at the pictures in glossy magazines, or watch Hollywood movies and admire how glamorous the women are? You may even wish you could be like them, if only in a small way.

Putting things into perspective, we don't necessarily always consider that it takes a lot of time and effort to look the way they do on camera – and even more patience and willpower (not to mention discipline) to maintain it. Although it may appear to come naturally, that probably couldn't be further from the truth. On the contrary; it takes a lot of hard work to look 'naturally beautiful'.

Everyone is beautiful in their own way. The secret is to make the most of what you have. It doesn't need to cost the earth, but it can take time – and, sometimes, a whole lot of effort.

It all starts with a decision. First, you have to want it – and not everybody does. So, make the decision to commit to feeling more gorgeous before you embark on any choices and actions to be more glamorous.

Start from the base up

Start from the base and work up from there. In this instance, the base is your skin. If you haven't done so already, begin with a healthy skin routine. As I mentioned in *Life Lessons from a 40 something…: For The Best Start In Life*, ensure you cleanse, tone and moisturise your face regularly. Include a frequent face mask, and exfoliate at least twice a week. This is crucial for achieving a polished look. Having a regular facial will also do wonders for your skin and help maintain its appearance. It has many benefits for your mind too, as it sets up the feel-good receptors in your brain. This shows self-love, helping you appreciate yourself for who you are. It can also be very relaxing, putting you in a calm and happy place. You should also pay attention to your body, again, exfoliating regularly and moisturising after you shower or bathe. Being glamorous means feeling good from head to toe.

Dress like you mean it

Next, dress like you meant it! For a purpose, not just because you find the easiest thing to pull out of your wardrobe. Take the time to consider your outfits; this is all part of caring for yourself. Clear away any clothes that are worn out or don't make you feel good anymore. You deserve to look and feel your best, including choices of what you wear. You are now at a prime time in life; gone are the days where you buy clothes that only last a week and just follow the trend. Now you can choose a few select pieces that are of a good quality and which can be incorporated into a variety of outfits, for various occasions.

Know your colours

Make the time to do your research and discover what colours bring out the best in you. If it helps, go shopping with a friend who is genuinely interested in helping you make the right choices. You could even hire a stylist to revolutionise your wardrobe. I did this once and it really helped me get excited about clothes again. I felt like a teenager once more. Hearing another person's views on what would look good on you can be an eye-opener. Sometimes, what we think won't work together, works together beautifully. I remember, in my days of working in retail, how good people felt when they tried on outfits that they thought would never suit them – and, suddenly, just one small suggestion from another and they felt amazing!

Take care of your hair

Taking care of your crowning glory is a must! Getting your hair done almost always works a as a quick pick-me-up. Experiment with styles and colours that bring out the best in you. Take care of the condition of your hair, too. I know how hard it can be to fit this in with our busy lives. But just conditioning your hair after shampooing can make a great deal of difference. Ask your hairdresser for advice, to assist you in making the most of your locks.

Polish up your make-up

Go through any make-up you have and get rid of anything that has expired. Wash any brushes and test out new make-up samples you may have been given. If you're stuck for ideas, try watching videos online; there are many tutorials you can follow, for tips and tricks. It's also worth noting that, just because you may have always done your make-up a certain way, it doesn't mean you can't experiment with new ideas. I know this because I've done it myself, although I also have a tendency to think I already know it all, since I've used make-up for years. It's true that there are some old tricks still used today, e.g. drawing eyeliner on your top lid, as well as along the base of the eye, for a more dramatic effect. There are other tricks to be learnt, and some may even save you time. As well as this, I have discovered there are many new products out there. For instance, we used to have to buy foundation and compact powder separately but now there are 'all in one' versions, which can be such a time-saver. So, just because you think you know it all, it doesn't mean you do! Things are always

135

evolving, especially in the worlds of make-up and fashion. Don't be afraid to experiment; you may even find it fun!

Feel glamorous

Feeling glamorous is a state of mind. If you feel good on the inside, it'll be reflected outwardly. Smile and radiate success, as you ooze glamour from every pore! Own it and allow yourself to have fun with this. Hire a photographer or get someone to take photos of you as you pose for the camera. This can be such a confidence-booster, with the added bonus that the photos remain a reminder of how glamorous and gorgeous you can be, especially when you look and feel like a million dollars.

Looking your best will help you to also feel your best. It has nothing to do with other people's opinions of you. Those will be more to do with them, than you. Even so, people don't – on the whole – like change and may, at first, express surprise at what they see. Disregard any unwelcome comments. Remember, there's no reason why they can't do the same as you. They may even be

136

wishing, secretly, that they had the courage to do what you are doing. Let this all glide over you, as you smile.

You'll very likely get to the point where you feel so good about yourself that you want to continue to feel that way! And that will inspire you to continue with the efforts you're making.

Keep going, Beautiful! Be the star of your own show, as you continue to add a touch of glamour to your life.

Fame

When I was younger, I used to dream of being a pop star. I used to admire stars like Duran Duran, Madonna and Prince – along with the jet-set lifestyles they led and all the attention and admiration they received. I used to whisper to myself that I would have the same, one day.

Upon reflection, I later realised that it wasn't so much their lives that I wanted for myself, after all. At a deeper level it wasn't just the attention I craved. In fact, even at just a basic

137

level, it was love that I wanted—or needed, to be more accurate.

When I was growing up, no-one ever dared mention that they wanted to be famous, for fear of being ridiculed – especially at school. I was a quiet person and whenever asked what I'd like to do, I used to say that I didn't know, or would mention a routine occupation. I didn't want to draw any outside attention to my real dream.

Nowadays, things have changed, however, and it tends to be okay to say you want to be famous. In fact it's quite the norm in many circles. There are countless celebrities who are 'famous for being famous' and having the time of their lives!

I often wonder if what they wanted was the same as what I wanted, when I was younger. I now realise that being – and feeling – loved isn't just something that people 'want'; it is a basic human need! We all need attention and to be loved, and to know that someone cares for us unconditionally. Everyone has a need to know that they are worthy and 'good enough'. I have also come to the conclusion that everyone likes to feel they are making a difference, however small. We each want to be significant in someone else's life.

Once I realised this, my whole outlook took on a whole new meaning. It transformed, from me being at the centre of my universe, to discovering ways in which I could make a difference to someone else – in other words, how I could be of greater service.

Those jet-set lifestyles we see portrayed are really only scratching the surface. When looking beneath, I realise that coming from a place of service, from the heart – and showing and sharing love through your work, your life and all that you do is what makes you extraordinary. In a way, it's what makes all of us, who do this, like pop stars!

You can be the star of your own show – and your own life. You can really make that difference, even if it's only in your own small area of the world – and even just from your own home.

Search inside, because inside all of us is a star waiting to come out.

Let your inner star shine bright!

CHAPTER 15

Dress for success

Dress for success

The way you dress speaks volumes and can
instantly establish you as a person of
authority, combined with effective
positioning. This includes your posture, how
you stand, the way you walk and how you sit
– which all help to pull your whole image
together.

Visualise your look

Before we begin with more details of the
practical side, let's run through a brief
visualisation you can use, to help set your
new look in motion:

- Close your eyes and imagine yourself
  as a successful, go-getting person who
  has everything she dreams of, in the
  palm of her hand.

- What does this feel like?

- What clothes are you wearing?

- Are you wearing jewellery? If so, what pieces are you wearing? Are they something sparkly or are they pearls?

- What perfume or scent can you smell?

- Are you smiling?

- What can you hear around you? For example, can you hear music, or chatting?

- How does looking this good make you feel, exactly? Let your imagination run; there is no limit to your potential! Tap into this moment.

- Open your eyes, as you smile to yourself, in glorious anticipation of what lies ahead for you.

Feel good? Great!

Now it's time to have some fun! Remember the clothes you were wearing in your visualisation? Let's bring them into reality.

Organise your clothes

First off, declutter your wardrobe. Only keep the clothes you love, as they make you feel good.

Being minimalist in your approach can alleviate problems in the future, especially if you have clothes bursting out of your wardrobe. Remember, lots of clutter equals lots of stress.

This is when a capsule wardrobe can come in handy. This means you have a set number of items that you can mix and match, including clothes for formal occasions, casual wear, sleepwear, sportswear and work wear. This is a useful habit to get into for, if and when you travel; it makes carrying your suitcase lighter too!

Hang your clothes up where you can; otherwise, fold them neatly. It's amazing how seeing everything in a neat, orderly fashion can make you feel calm, and that you have it altogether – thus easing stress.

If you can, try and choose the clothes you're wearing in advance, especially if planning an

143

event or night out. Preparing in advance takes away any angst along the, 'I've got nothing to wear' lines.

Getting organised means you know what clothes you have. It avoids you buying duplicates – or ones that look very similar – and prepares you for buying new clothes.

Time to go shopping

Let the shopping begin! Don't just go for items you usually buy and are comfortable in, though. Be open to change, perhaps even adding a splash of colour here and there. A different colour can work wonders; it lifts your mood and boosts morale, especially on a rainy day.

Something to bear in mind, when shopping, is to try to buy pieces that can go towards making multiple outfits. For example, a black skirt can be worn with several tops and to lots of occasions, a white top can be combined with lots of coloured skirts, trousers and jeans.

Look for pieces that closely match what you had in mind. Have a browse online, or look through magazines. These don't necessarily have to be expensive clothes; it's okay to buy economical pieces, until you're ready to splash out on investment pieces that will last longer. This is where a 'cost-per-wear' formula comes in handy:

$$\frac{Price\ of\ garment}{Number\ of\ times\ to\ wear} = Cost - per - wear$$

For example, a blouse priced at £25, which you plan to wear twice a month for eight months, would be calculated as:

£25 (Price) ÷ 16 (2 x 8 = sum of times you plan to wear it) = £1.56 (cost-per-wear).

A coat priced at £350, which you plan to wear daily (thirty days) for three months a year, that is estimated to last for five years, can be calculated as:

£350 (Price) ÷ 450 (30 x 3 x 5 = sum of times you plan to wear it) = £0.78 (cost- per- wear).

This makes you look at your choices in a whole new light, and will prove more economical in the long run. Think of quality over quantity.

Style yourself for success

If you are dressing to create a good impression, such as a special occasion or other, important event, ask yourself, "What does this outfit say about me?" This is very helpful for when you are going to an event and don't wish to stand out too much. Check the dress code and dress accordingly. You want to wear something smart but perhaps also something that you don't want to spend the whole-time fidgeting and feeling self-conscious about. This is in contrast to when you are going out for the evening and want to get glammed up! You can afford to get out your sequins and pearls for nights out, none of which will look out of place.

On the other hand, if you are going out and about during the day or are at home, get as casual as you want to. Comfort is the key here, so that you are able to move around with ease and feel relaxed.

Don't be afraid to try something on that you wouldn't choose, normally. Just because it doesn't look great on a hanger doesn't mean you won't look good in it! With more than two decades of experience in the fashion industry, there have been many times when I've suggested a dress that, at first glance, looked plain on the hanger. As soon as someone tried it on, however, I would see their face light up. They were delighted at how good it looked on them and how amazing they felt.

While it's good to know what colours suit you and bring out the best in your appearance, it can also an eye-opener to try out different colours. You may be pleasantly surprised at the results! Colours give you a wonderful boost when you are feeling down, transforming your energy levels almost immediately.

Finishing touches

Don't forget the shoes, of course! Try on different pairs and aim for ones that look good as well as giving a level of comfort, if possible. There's nothing worse than feet being in agony, with blisters rubbing up the back of your heel! Nor wearing shoes that are so much higher than you're used to, that it looks like you're hobbling around

147

everywhere. If you are, indeed, planning to wear higher than normal heels, for a special event, allow yourself enough time to practise wearing them beforehand. Having a full dress rehearsal will help alleviate all kinds of unwarranted situations and unnecessary stress.

Remember, too, handbags or clutch bags – and, of course jewellery and accessories that help to pull the whole look together. Complement your attire! It's the finishing touches that hold the real magic and give your look that certain, 'Je ne sais quoi'.

Now the fun part! This is the bit where you get to put everything together. Try on the clothes and 'mix and match' with shoes and accessories.

Have fun with experimenting!

Brand new you

You should be feeling like a 'brand new you', by now. This is so good for morale, helping you to feel as though you can accomplish anything!

Aim to do things that make you feel brand new and that will lift your spirits more often. These may include getting your hair done, having your nails painted and having a regular facial. You could even consider hiring a make-up artist, to give you a makeover and some helpful tips on how to maintain your fresh look.

Show off

Give yourself permission to show off your revived and amazing new look. You deserve to, especially when you look so jaw-droppingly gorgeous! Are you feeling brave enough to do more? Why not book a photo session? This can be so much fun and a perfect way of celebrating 'you'. As an added bonus, you can treasure the photos, which will act as a reminder of how glamorous you truly are – when you allow yourself to live to your fullest potential.

CHAPTER 16

Unlock your gorgeousness

Love how you look

Now it's time to tap into that inner beauty of yours. Yes, I'm talking to you not the person behind you or next to you! I mean *you*.

Take a moment and look at yourself in the mirror; not in a fault-finding, 'My hips are too wide...', kind of way, but in a, 'I love the shape of my legs; my stomach looks amazing...', kind of way. You know what I mean?

Next, think of a time when you felt fantastic! It could be recently or in the more distant past. If it helps, grab some photos of yourself from when you were younger and know you felt gorgeous. Look at one of those photos and try to recapture how you felt.

What was happening at that time? If you were dressing up for a party, feel the excitement in the air; notice the energy and any anticipation of things to come. Were you playing music to help get in the mood? What were you wearing? What colour was your lipstick? How did you wear your hair? What perfume did you have on?

Make this as vivid as you can; so much so, that all you have to do is look at the photo to prompt you – and, suddenly, all those feelings come flooding back. I expect you are feeling great! Now, it's time to anchor the feelings, so you can continue to tap into them any time you want to. While you're drifting down memory lane, then, place your middle finger and your thumb together and really hone in on those feelings. This sets everything in motion, triggering your memory and activating all the good feelings in you. This way, any time you want to tap into and rekindle the happy memory, you can just press your finger and thumb together and 'Voila!' You will be back to a time when you felt gorgeous.

Use your senses

Another thing you can do involves using your physical senses. For instance, if you spray some perfume on your wrist, this will serve as a reminder. You will suddenly feel revived. Because you felt gorgeous back then, you are likely to do so again. Listening to music can also help. You could play a song that makes you feel good or makes you want to strut your stuff, we all have at least one!

Borrow inspiration

If, for some reason, you're unable to recall a time when you felt gorgeous – and if you haven't got any photos – then you can always 'borrow' such a memory from someone else and use it for your inspiration. For example, you could get a photo of a celebrity you admire and 'play' at being them, for a few minutes. Really get into the role. Imagine you were them having your photo taken. Pretend you're wearing their clothes and stepping into their shoes, for the day. If you feel like it, even practise speaking like them. It's all in the name of fun, so you may as well enjoy yourself in this process! Children can do this

153

kind of thing very easily. For the rest of us, it's just that, as we get older, we lose the ability and seem to care too much about what others think of us. That's a shame, because we can lose so much in the process of being too serious at times. Now's the time to release your inhibitions and really get into that groove with it all.

You may even find it easier to play the role of someone else, sometimes, as opposed to drawing from your own experience. This could be because it's easier to remain detached and free from any past emotions that may come up. That's okay – in this instance, anyway, because we are focusing on you loving the way you look.

Another thing that may come up is that some people feel a little foolish and will go so far as to play down their attractiveness, to 'fit in' with the crowd. While this may seem rational, at the time, it won't do you any favours when it comes to developing your self-esteem. So, tell yourself now, "I am gorgeous!" Now, say it again – and, this time, say it like you *really* mean it. "I am *gorgeous!*" Now, smile at yourself. Hold on to this moment and really believe it. In future, say this regularly to yourself. Remember, the more often you can say it aloud, the faster you will be able to really get into the energy of it. That is when you'll be ready to truly unlock your gorgeousness.

Really own this, now. Even see it in the way you walk. Enjoy yourself! Inject gorgeousness into your every move. Walk like you truly believe that you are beautiful – because you are.

Sparkles and sunshine

Let yourself sparkle from the inside out. Indulge in the magnificent you! When you are brimming with joy on the inside, you can't help but overflow with happiness on the outside. It shows in everything you do; from the moment your feet touch the floor, in the morning, to waving, 'Hello', at a friend during the day, to then ending your day with a smile placed firmly on your lips.

There's something quite magical about being in a state of grace and filled with abundance.

It's having that resounding assurance that you just know everything is as it should be. And it's all happening at a time that is just right for you. Having this wonderful wisdom makes you more alluring. It sets you apart from others – and it's what makes you, *'you'*.

Shine your light brightly and boldly for all the world to see. Let it radiate out to others. Allow it to overflow in sparkling bubbles of delight, as you move towards a brighter vision of love. Be filled with acceptance of your own, silky-soft demeanour, wrapped in the strong powerhouse that you are. Stand tall and embrace the pillar of light within you.

Let your life be filled with sparkles and sunshine, as you look towards a tomorrow that's bursting with promise.

You deserve to be beautiful and – above all – to feel amazing. No more hiding in the shade for you, Sunshine! It's time for you to step out of the shadows, put on that wide-brimmed hat and be *fabulous*.

CHAPTER 17

Fortune

Learning about money

When I had just started working, at the beginning of almost every month, when I went to the cash machine for money, it would say I was *in credit*. Then, after I'd take out only a small amount, it would say I was *in debit*. I could never understand this back then. I didn't understand about being overdrawn. The slip that used to come with the cash never carried much detail. I recall being annoyed with myself, for not being able to make sense of it all.

Back then, I worked in retail and was only taking home approximately four hundred pounds per month, which wasn't really much at all. Luckily, I was living with my parents at the time, although I still had to pay them rent and this took most of the money for the month.

I never thought about getting a credit card; the idea just never entered my head. I used to save up for absolutely everything I wanted. Back then, music played a big part in my life and I used to save up for musical equipment. I remember, particularly, saving up for a P.A. system and going into the shop to buy it. I paid with cash and will never forget how heavy the equipment was. My sister and I had to lift it and carry it back home; it was far too heavy for two, very slim girls. It's a wonder we ever got it home without causing damage to the equipment, or ourselves! But thankfully we did. I always paid in cash back then and – to be honest – wasn't quite sure how cards worked.

Later on, after the break-up of my marriage, I found myself as a single parent, with numerous store and credit cards. At one point I even had three jobs, as I was determined to provide for my family. Luckily, I had the support of my mother-in-law, who looked after my son while I went out to work. It was tough, but we got through it.

I came to the realisation that I had to transform my money pattern, fast! Quite frankly, if I wasn't going to do it, there was nobody else to support me. I was the main breadwinner and something had to change – not least because I had a son to think of. Funnily enough it was during this same year that I started a savings account for my son, since I didn't want him to go through what did. I wanted him to be in a stronger position than I was! So, I began doing things differently. I started finding ways to bring in and attract more money into my life.

If you are in a similar situation, realise that things *can* change. It is never too late to change your money patterns. Yes, you, too, can learn all about money; it's really not as hard as a lot of people think it is.

Fast forward a few years and I got a job in a bank where I had intense training. I learnt, swiftly, all the ins and outs of how to manage a bank account. I became so good at it that I didn't even realise that I had begun to find it a whole lot easier – I was enjoying it, too! I enjoyed it so much, in fact, that I soon got promoted. I became a personal account manager, where my job involved helping others to manage their bank accounts, all day long. I enjoyed this immensely; it all came so naturally to me. It then seemed almost as though my younger days, when I didn't have a clue, had happened to a stranger and not to me!

Becoming debt-free

There came a point when I was determined to clear all my debts. I read a lot about the law of attraction and visualisation. I used to spend my lunchtime sitting in a bookshop, getting immersed in those types of books. I started saying regular affirmations and using crystals. I even experimented with a little Feng Shui. In my mission to be debt-free, I regularly visualised my credit card statement balances being reduced to £0.00. I also worked very hard. As my job was very target-driven, I used to make sure I achieved those targets. I worked really hard and attained pay increases; bonuses were a big help, too, as we would get a bonus every quarter. I remember being at a manager's meeting, where everyone was talking about the latest watch or car that they'd bought themselves. I kept quiet, because I had used my bonus to help pay off my credit cards. By then, I had transferred balances so that I was paying zero interest. I took pleasure in watching those credit balances getting lower and lower. Then, one day, I held my credit card statement in my hand and jumped for joy, when I saw that my visualisation had come true. The balance finally showed £0.00!

After that, I closed all the other credit card accounts and kept only one, for emergencies. If I did have to use it, I would make sure that I cleared the balance within the given 30 days, so that I wouldn't incur any interest.

I am living proof that it's possible to become debt-free. I was also happy that I was in a position to help others befriend their finances and take control, so that they too could be much happier in their lives.

I also couldn't believe the amount of people who were too afraid to even look at their bank statements, let alone talk about their financial situation. After I spent time helping them and explaining things to them, they always left much happier, with a better understanding. They eventually gained the confidence to manage their own accounts and watch them flourish. I loved seeing the positive changes this brought and the difference in their demeanour.

If you are in this position, take heart, because there's no mystery in money. You, too, can manage your finances and build wealth. It all starts with wanting to *change* your financial situation; once you've got this, you are ready to go.

Track your money

Firstly, you need to track what's going in and out of your account, on a monthly basis.

Here's an example:

INCOME	FIXED OUTGOINGS	
2000	Rent 1000	1st
1100 – (total outgoings)	Gas 60	4th
900 left for the month	Water 40	8th
	Total: 1100	

Next:
- Write down your expected income on the left and fixed outgoings on the right.

- Subtract your outgoings from your income, on the left.

- Each time you spend any more money, subtract it from the number that is left over on the left column.

Here's an example of how that would work:

INCOME	FIXED OUTGOINGS	
2000	Rent 1000	1st
1100 – (total outgoings)	Gas 60	4th
900 left for the month	Water 40	8th
- 40 (gift)		
860 left		
- 30 (sweater)		
830 left	Total: 1100	

Be sure to track everything you spend. I also find it useful to write down whatever I have bought; that way, I can easily see where my money is going. This is useful for assessing and tweaking spending habits, if necessary.

This may take some getting used to, but, once you've done it a few times, it'll get easier.

Make a budget

You then need to make a budget. Budgets are not about limiting how we live. On the contrary, a budget will give you more freedom to do the things you want, in a way that won't bring you into debt. You can budget for fun activities, too. Write down all your regular payments on this sheet; remember to include even the littlest things. You may start to see a pattern emerging and be able to trim down things you don't really need.

Now go through your direct debits and standing orders and cancel or amend any that you no longer need. There may, for instance, be a few where you no longer use the related services, or had just forgotten to cancel.

165

Changing them will help easily conserve some of your income.

Consolidate your debts. If you have high interest credit cards, do what I did and transfer them to a lower interest card or, ideally, a zero-interest card.

While on the subject of direct debits and standing orders, see if you can change the dates on them, so that they all come out around a similar time of the month. I tend to have mine go out on the 1st of each month, but you may want to have yours towards the end. Find out which works better for you. The idea is that you don't miss paying any of them, as well as trying to avoid overdraft fees, or keeping those to a minimum.

Check your utility bills and see if you can switch any to a cheaper provider. Don't be afraid to do so. As I have always said, 'The money is better in your pocket than in theirs!'

Once you have done this for a few months, you should begin to see your account transform, for the better. Remember, you can always seek advice, whether that may be online or by going to chat to someone who can assist you. There are plenty of people out there who can help, so don't feel embarrassed to ask. Everyone has to start somewhere — I certainly did!

Shop smart

Shopping is a big money absorber, for many people. Before making a purchase, ask yourself these questions:

- Do I really need it?

- Can I save up for it?

- Do I need it right now?

- What's it worth to me? (i.e. time or money. Most things cost you your time or your money. Do you value these enough to exchange either or both of them for this purchase?)

Bargains can also be a selling ploy. Ask yourself, 'Is it really a bargain?' If you think it is, then go back over the first question of whether you really need it – and so on,

through relevant questions from the rest of
the list.

Build your wealth

If you want to create a fortune, you need to
begin by building your wealth. This can take
time, so a little patience is required. Start by
putting away ten percent of available income
in a savings account and try not to touch it.
Before you know it, this will build up to a nice
sum and, when it does, you can either buy
something or put a portion of it away into a
higher interest account. It always helps to
have an end goal in mind. What would you
love to save up for?

Investing a small amount is a great way of
compounding the capital itself plus the
interest you receive on it. This will
accumulate, like magic, if you allow it to
grow. Read books and carry out research
before investing. I am not a financial advisor,
and you need to do that research, as 'stocks
can go down as well as up', as they say. Don't
rely on this money, as there is an element of
risk involved. Only invest an amount you can
afford to lose. Having said that, although this

is not for the faint-hearted, there are some terrific gains to be made.

Give back

Tithe. In the bible it recommends to tithe ten percent of your income. This could go to a charity or a cause that you hold dear to your heart. This is a part of humanitarianism, as it is always nice to share with others who need our help. Do this from a place of giving and with a grateful heart, as helping others is a reward in itself.

Just start

The main thing about growing your wealth is to begin. It doesn't matter how small an amount you start with, because it's more about the habits that you make. In time, they can build upon each other and compound. Before you know it, your wealth will build and things won't seem as bleak as perhaps they once did. So, just start – and see what happens.

Plant those seeds of success, today, so that you may reap the rewards from them in the future.

CHAPTER 18

Excitement

Craving excitement

From when I was a teenager, right up to my early thirties, there were times when I craved excitement. I was full of restless energy and needed to move fast and make things happen. I didn't realise that this could also attract things to happen a little too fast sometimes. Some of these were thrilling experiences, while others weren't quite so welcome. At times I played the drama queen and demanded attention. At other times, I required solitude, feeling the need to do my own thing. It went from one extreme to another, like a real-life rollercoaster. I experienced the highs and expected the lows. I was full of passion, purpose and determination. Headstrong and driven, nothing and no-one could control me, or, indeed, stop me.

As I grew older – and became more sensible – I no longer felt the need for drama in my life. I had learnt from past experiences that what I needed now was so different from what I'd wanted before. These days, I yearn for peace and to feel comfortable. I like the quiet life and steer clear of people and situations that tend to provoke drama. I value peace and find that different things bring me joy. I no longer need the hustle, bustle and fast pace that I once did. I prefer to take things slower and go at my own speed.

I do still get excited about things. I just don't need the drama that can sometimes come with excitement. I love feeling excited in a positive way, one that lifts the spirit and raises energy levels. Excitement enables high vibrations that surround us and makes us feel good. Excitement can be infectious and so encourages others to also feel part of the happy vibe.

I now realise that excitement can mean different things to different people. While someone might find climbing a tall mountain exhilarating, another person may prefer being surrounded by animals at a safari park. One person could prefer to go kick-boxing, whilst another may enjoy birdwatching.

Find excitement on your terms, regardless of what others may think of it. You are never too old to get excited about things! Give yourself permission to get excited about your life. You have the power to make it as exciting as you want it to be. Enjoy the thrill.

Finding balance

I understand how important it is to have balance in your life. A little excitement now and then, with a little down time, helps to sustain and maintain a happy life. It keeps you on the right track and helps to avoid the lows. That way, it's not so much of a rollercoaster ride, as a calm and purposeful journey. You can ride the waves but also enjoy the calmness. A little bit of both goes a long way.

Grounding

I have learnt that it is beneficial to re-group and keep grounded. This helps to avoid

173

exhaustion, or the burnout that often occurs with life's high spots. Grounding will help you to stay calm and maintain focus, as you go about your day. It will help your inner strength, which is an essential part of supporting your general wellbeing. By not getting caught up in all the commotion, feeling lost among dizzy heights, you will feel centred and able to tap into your inner peace. This will help you feel whole and solid.

Eternal optimism

Being optimistic is more than feeling positive while others are feeling down. It's being able to tap into the energy of abundance when circumstances appear bleak. It's about being relentless in your pursuit for success and happiness. It's having faith when nobody else 'gets it'. It's having unprecedented love for yourself and others, when other people around you aren't being supportive. It's the 'knowing', whilst feeling misunderstood. Stay unshakeable in your passion and in your urgency for the truth.

A technique that can enable you to feel good is reframing, or re-positioning, an event that happened in the past, so that you are able to move forward with your life. This has been explained in more detail in Chapter 11, 'Master Reframing'.

It is optimism that marks the difference between the warrior and the defeated. It is hope that triumphs over failure. Having optimism makes it possible to love and endure tribulations – and it is love that conquers all.

Eternal optimism is an expression of love in its finest form. It keeps us going, when it feels easier to walk away. Let your optimism shine through, while others stare at the dark. Carry your light and let it lead the way, so that you can share it with others who have gone astray.

Fun

It's okay to have a little (or even a lot of) fun, along the way. Just because you are at a different stage of your life doesn't mean that the fun has to stop; it may just come in an unexpected way. Rather than having tight schedules and constant deadlines, leave enough flexibility in your day-to-day routine to allow for fun activities. Laughter is the best way to keep your soul happy, whilst your mind is occupied with happy surprises. Not everything has to be planned; this is part of the joy of living.

You can have fun with loved ones, or even by yourself. Look for opportunities and inject as much fun into your daily life as you possibly can. The world will seem much brighter when you look at it from a lighter place in your heart. This is a place where you are free from judgement and the need to perform, or to do what is expected of you. Try, instead, to enjoy your life as much as you can. Enjoying what you do keeps things interesting and keeps you feeling young.

Life can be so exciting and fun! Let go of the drama and get excited for the right reasons. It's time to get excited in such a way that you are bursting with sunshine and happiness – in your heart and in your soul. Make today a great day to be alive!

CHAPTER 19

Freedom

Moment of clarity

To have complete freedom means being without limits. This includes those that you place on yourself – and those you believe other people have placed on you. This is quite a rare state, simply because we have all, at one time or another, blamed other people for why we haven't achieved something or gone somewhere. It's our way of excusing ourselves for not accomplishing things, including casual ideas, as well as bigger goals that we've always wanted to fulfil.

It's when we start taking responsibility for our actions and efforts that we begin to see things as they really are, however. It's a little like removing tinted glasses, when a truer, clearer view appears. Perhaps this is just what we have been afraid of, all along! That is, to discover that we're the real reason why we have held back in the past. This is not always easy to digest; it may be easier to blame others for our actions – or lack of actions.

This is not the time to start beating yourself up over anything, however. Think of it, instead, as a revelation, as well as a sign that you can do something about it. After all, what is seen cannot be unseen.

Feel

Take a deep breath and really feel what you have always wanted to feel. Notice the elation in your body as you can finally unleash what your heart and soul have been asking – almost begging – you to do, all along. You do not require anyone's permission to live the life you have always dreamed of; you never really have done. Even though you may have blamed your parents or others for a long time, there comes a stage in life where you need to own it and, instead, step into the shoes that were meant for you – and you alone.

Stay wild

Think back to a time when life was filled with hope and possibility; a time when you truly believed you could do whatever you wanted to do. Meet the changemaker in you! You felt like nobody would ever stand in your way, because you could make the impossible, possible. How did you feel?

Did you act on your impulses? If you'd wanted to go and hang out by the beach, would you have simply jumped into a car – perhaps with your beau at the time? Would you have taken off with the wind in your hair, singing your heart out to the music that was playing – laughing, without a care in the world? Or maybe you preferred stillness and took pleasure in being the quiet rebel?

No matter the case, that was a time when you felt wild and free. It was the time when you were celebrating life in its truest form. Letting your inner child out once in a while, in joyous celebration, is okay; it's great for your mind and spirit. It reminds you that you are alive!

Do this as often as you can. You're not being irresponsible, as long as you're not harming anybody else. Do it for yourself. Giving yourself a boost of unexpected joy does wonders for your morale and gives you a burst of energy, which can feel quite exhilarating.

Allow yourself to return to the innocence of your youth – a time when things didn't matter quite as much, because you could just live in the moment and get excited by the now.

Innocence is a virtue. Remember your inner child and stay curious about everything you do. This may mean visiting a place you've always wanted to visit, or playing loud music, perhaps dancing away to it. Allow yourself to indulge in the days that have passed; this will bring renewed vitality to your time ahead.

Remember your yesterdays. Clothed in the wisdom of time, stay you and stay wild!

Enjoy your sense of adventure

You don't always have to have everything planned out to the smallest detail. Sometimes you just have to go with it and see where the road leads you. Keep yourself open to opportunities and keep your mind flexible. Be willing to try new adventures, regardless of how scary they may at first seem. With a sense of adventure and a happy heart, who knows what is on the horizon!

Lay your fears to rest and embrace the excitement of the unexpected. Miracles often happen when we least anticipate them. Allow yourself to feel butterflies, as you leap into the unknown with a completely carefree soul.

Just making the decision to do what you've always dreamt of will make you feel so much better. Go where you've always wanted to go; be who you've always wanted to be and try on the lifestyle you've continuously wanted.

Notice the changes in you. How do you feel? Describe the sensory experience; how does this taste? Take a look at the bigger picture; what can you see? Can you hear laughter, as you thoroughly enjoy being in this moment?

It's time to wake-up to the life of your dreams! Feel the wind beneath your wings and embrace the spirit within you that's urging you to go on and fulfil your destiny. There's no longer a need to pretend, waiting until you're ready. The time has come to take off the veil you've been hiding under; the one that felt so comfortable for so long. Shed the memories that no longer serve you. Release those anxious thoughts that have been holding you back. No limits are allowed where you are going; you are so done with those!

Live like there's no tomorrow

Don't be afraid. Let your fear fuel your vision, as you drive forward with strength and vigour, towards your true calling. This is who you were meant to be. You may not have known it then, but you surely do now! Bring on the challenges that you are going to overcome. You did so before and can do so again. You have *so* got this! Believe in yourself and the possibilities of what can be, countering any discouragement about what lies ahead. The promise of a brighter tomorrow is often preceded by a heavy heart, but this can be turned around – in more ways than anyone could possibly imagine.

Remove the chains that have held you down and allow yourself to cheer with joy, as you taste the freedom ahead with an open spirit running through your hair. Live like there's no tomorrow, without the worries of yesteryear. This is your time to shine the brightest you have ever thought possible. Don't be afraid to shine so bright that others can no longer look away from the brilliance, bursting out of every cell and pore of your body.

Let your light beam for all the world to see, for what lies within you is more powerful than any negativity has ever been. Trust in the whispers that you tried not to hear, before – and in the visions you pretended you could not see. Trust also in the words you felt too afraid to tell. These have all led to this moment in time. Words do not matter to a song that has been sung; the tune has already been played on a plane far beyond.

Your true essence

Tap into your true essence, a spirit that's your power source, held deep within you. As you set upon your path, on a journey unknown,

183

feel the excitement surge you onward; it can empower you to go beyond, to any place you have never been before. Seek out that place you have always dreamt of, the one where your soul feels at home. This doesn't have to be planned; it could be a voyage without destination – just believe, and go with it. Live in the flow that has its own purpose, even if it doesn't make sense right now. All will be revealed at the right time. The heart needs no reason. Remember that logic sometimes shades the truth from a quizzical nature. Allow yourself to proceed without rhyme or reason. Take the first step, and the rest will follow.

Embrace the freedom to be yourself – and watch the magic happen!

CHAPTER 20

Growth

Growth

One thing you can be certain of in life is that everything is continuously changing. This is part of life and inevitable, especially where you want to improve in positive ways. Even in technology, innovation is a much-needed ingredient, in the effort to streamline, improve efficiency and achieve progress for the future.

Without growth, we'd become stagnant and perhaps not feel as motivated or excited about the future. Things would seem mundane and might even become a little boring. We don't want that, especially when it comes to leading a fabulous life!

Growth can be exhilarating and fun. It brings about an energy of expansion that can light us up and make us feel like we can do anything. Allow yourself to go with this and explore the new perspective it offers. It can bring you to new heights, ones that will send you dizzy with delight, as you discover your full potential. There's a world of possibilities awaiting you!

Stand firm, on a solid foundation

First you need to stand firm, on a solid foundation, which you can use as a springboard for success. Ensure you are in a positive state of mind. Mindset is key to almost anything in life and is particularly useful before you are about to embark on any journey of discovery and adventure. So, let's get you from this quiet, standing point, to taking quantum strides of success.

Get clear on your vision

Ask yourself what it is that you want to achieve. Visualise it into existence. You could begin with putting together a vision board. This can be quite fun, as it brings you back to your younger days, when you weren't afraid of asking for what you wanted. I remember, as a child, going through home catalogues and turning down the corners of the pages to show what I wanted. It was a little like a child having a wish list for Christmas; a list for a future shopping spree. I can remember how excited I felt, just at the thought of getting those toys and playing with them. Except that, for you, in the here and now, this isn't just make-believe. Now that you are all grown-up, there's a greater chance you could actually get the things you want; the main difference being that your choice of 'toys' has probably changed.

In your mission to achieve your wish list, keep your eyes peeled for images and quotes that identify with the lifestyle you desire. When you find them, cut them out or save them on your phone, laptop, computer etc. Gather them together so you can create a collage. Whether you do this by hand or virtually doesn't matter; the idea is to get a vision in your mind of what you'd like to achieve. Look at your vision board regularly; it serves as a reminder of your intention. This is a necessary step, as you start creating the life of your dreams. Once you have the vision set in your mind, you may start to feel your spirit rise within you, already. This is just the beginning, so get ready – your potential is just around the corner!

Knowledge is your superpower

This is when the work begins, but don't let that put you off. Learning can be fun! It's not like when you were at school and had little choice of the topics you had to learn. This time around, you are calling the shots; you get to choose what you enjoy and what you'd like to learn. Don't worry. As I said in *Life Lessons from a 40 something…: For The Best Start In Life*, 'Everything can be learnt'. This time around, there's the added beauty of the internet, which can be a wonder in itself. You have the world at your fingertips. You just have to open up your mind to that treasure trove of knowledge and everything will begin to fall into place – just like that. Okay, maybe not *just like that*, but you get the picture. It's easier than you may think; just begin, and see what unfolds. And remember, you *are* allowed to have fun while you learn!

Go ahead and see what you fancy. Do you want to get creative and take a workshop? Or stimulate your mind with a course? Do you even want to go so far as getting that degree you've always wanted to go after? Don't let your age put you off; it's never too late to learn. Newspaper reports say that now, more than ever, people over the age of sixty are studying for degrees and loving life. Education doesn't have to stop at the school or college gates. We are learning all the time. Knowledge can often be shared with others, too, given the right permissions. You may want to add value to your clients, family and friends, or perhaps teach students, even. There are so many opportunities wide open to you. If it makes you feel good, go do it!

Feed your curiosity

Think back to when you were a child and were filled with wonder and curiosity. I can recall countless times, when I asked my mother, "Mum, why does this...?" or "Mum, how come that...?" I wanted to know *everything*, especially why things were the way they were. Tap into that same curiosity that you had as a child. It is this thirst for knowledge that will keep you going.

189

Move forward in happy curiosity and feed the hunger to want to know more. This is the same hunger that drives you in your hunt for success. Refuse to be satisfied with 'just getting by' and with things being average, unless you are happy as you are. If you're not, recognise where you want more; the wanting will lead to action-taking, inevitably resulting in success.

People are often driven to get to the top of their chosen field because they don't feel satisfied with what they have; usually, it's because they want more out of life. What is it that you want? What drives you? Let your passion guide you to a path you truly love.

Be a creative explorer of the truth within

You are a fascinating creature! You have so much going for you, as you'll see, if you can only take the time to dive in and really gaze upon the beauty that you are. I don't just mean externally, either; I mean right down to your very core. Take the time to explore your hidden depths; here's where the inner, superhero lies within you. Envisage your highest self. Watch her grow into her full potential. Let the creative explorer within you arise, and watch her soar; this will reveal the true magic of you!

Wisdom

You have a special gift to offer; a gift that can't be bought. You have something that you can bring to the table. Your own experience matters. It is extensive and full of wonderful memories that can serve you well if you allow them to. Your wisdom is what defines you and sets you apart from others. Share your wisdom with other people; it is the most valuable gift there is and you'll always be remembered for it. While others may be flapping around you, you can remain calm and quiet, poised in the knowledge of life and grounded in the wisdom you've gained. Be a rock for others. Let your legacy live on, down the ages, through the wisdom you bring.

Expansion

Enjoy your newfound energy, filled with a sense of expansion. This will attract like-minded people to you and those with similar qualities; people who hunger for growth and feel empowered to build a new, improved way a life. You are helping to create a place where restless souls can come together in happy contentment, and excitement for life. When new faces unite, energies collide. Before you know it, such bursts of positive force can lead to a whole explosion of positivity and promise – in this world where nothing stands still. So, let yourself fly high, and continue to soar – just because you can.

CHAPTER 21

Drive

Why?

Why do you do the things you do? What is the main reason? When you know the reason behind what you do and why you do it, this serves as a springboard to your success. People tend to be either driven towards something or repelled away from a situation, person or group of people.

For instance, one man, who was brought up experiencing poverty, used to watch his mother scraping coins together, to buy a loaf of bread. He wore hand-me-downs, which his mother sewed and repaired, in an effort to give pieces of clothing new leases of life. He watched, as his classmates at school got all the latest toys and wore the latest fashions; he bowed his head down, comparing what he was wearing. He remembered how he felt, especially on the day when he got teased for having a hole in his trousers. Recalling his pain, he vowed that, when he was older, he'd be able to afford the latest fashions; he would not be worrying about money because he would have plenty of it. And so that man set his intention for success and wealth. For him, his 'Why?' was to move away from poverty and towards wealth.

As another example, a woman wanted to move to the country, to a slower pace of life. She wanted to go to a place where there would be a lot of space and fewer people around. She also wanted more freedom, and time to spend with her children; she wanted to raise them in a happier environment. So, she set up a business, making cupcakes. At first she made them for just a few people to enjoy. After receiving feedback, with people saying how delicious the cakes were, she began selling them at local churches, fairs and table-top sales. Orders came in thick and fast, so much so, that she had to rent premises and hire staff to take over making the cakes. What started out as a humble, little cupcake quickly evolved into something so much bigger than she had ever imagined possible.

All the while, the woman held her dream in her heart – the dream of moving to a big house in the country. As her profits increased, so did her savings. One day, she bought that big house in the country and she and her family couldn't have been happier! They even got some chickens, cows and horses, as they were surrounded by acres of rolling fields. Her dream had become her reality.

I have always been naturally driven, although my reasons have often changed. When I was a teenager, I remember taking part in a talent contest with my band. This was partly for a little fame, but mostly because I wanted the people around me to take the band seriously and realise that we weren't just messing around – that we had talent. We rehearsed like crazy! I'll admit, I was rather fastidious in my approach. I wanted everything to be 'just right' and took this out on the other members, who perhaps didn't put in quite as much effort as me. Having said that, they did all come through in the end. What helped was that we remembered the reason why we wanted to succeed, which kept us going. Fortunately, we did experience success, to the extent that people used to come up to me in the streets nearby and ask for my autograph. We even started a fan club; our first fan was from Wales. We eventually went our separate ways, as we wanted different things, but I still look back with fond memories.

Your 'Why', the reason behind why you want to achieve something, will help you when things don't seem possible, or the road ahead looks bleak. Like a flame in your heart, it will keep going, just as long your intention is there. In times of doubt, remember your 'Why'.

Be purposeful

Be purposeful, in your pursuit of success. Keep your goal at the forefront of your mind and do something towards it regularly – even if only a small step. It's the collection of tiny steps that can end up making big leaps toward achieving what you want.

Draw up a plan of action; just doing this can have a profound effect on making things happen. Suddenly, everything will appear more doable; once you start thinking that it is within your reach, you are more likely to take action. The prospect of achieving your goal turns out to be closer than you first thought.

Ambition

Ambition is not a dirty word! There have been many soap operas, particularly in the eighties, that have portrayed women with ambition as cold, heartless creatures; as those who would do anything in their mission for power and success. While the majority of men were the heads of business and involved in large corporations, back then, this isn't the case now. Times are changing. It's okay for you to be ambitious.

Whilst I've always been very ambitious, I'll admit that there have been occasions when I played this side of me down, for fear of being ridiculed or, even worse, laughed at! I went to an all-girls school. I remember, during one lesson, the teacher went around the class asking what everyone wanted to do when they left school. Most of the girls said things like a clerk, an accountant, a teacher, etc. When it came to me, although I was positively bursting to tell people what I wanted to do, I

197

didn't do so. Instead of saying, 'A songwriter', I said something like, 'A botanist'. I still wanted to stand out, but not too much – out of fear that the whole class would laugh at me.

Nowadays, I'm pleased to say it's a lot easier to tell others what you want to do, without negative repercussions. There are many children who want to be TV personalities, singers, musicians, etc.

Don't be afraid to be ambitious. It is fun and exciting. It makes an interesting conversation-starter, too.

Stay hungry

Stay hungry for success; absorb it into your being. Be eager in your pursuit for it and let yourself get excited by the prospect of it. The anticipation and excitement you feel will empower you to take great strides forward, in your mission. This will be the fuel that keeps you going.

Strive to be your best

Strive for excellence. Master all the skills that you can, to be the best you can be. Focus on optimum performance and put your heart and soul into it. Aim to deliver the best possible service you can. In this way, your impeccable standards will reinforce your integrity to others and you'll reap the rewards.

Passion

When you speak, do it from your heart. Mean everything you say. If you feel strongly about a topic, express it in a way that's positive and purposeful. Having good intentions outweighs many things. If you feel you don't know much about a topic, don't let that stop you from voicing your opinion. Enthusiasm and passion connect to others faster; they're often more effective than detailed facts.

Be awesome

You don't have to do things the same way that others do. You can find your own way and pave your own path. How you say or do something is unique to you and to be

199

admired. Your take on things may be different to someone else's and that's okay, as we all have something to bring to the table. Stop worrying about the masses. Just like there are many paths to success, there are many stories to share – including yours. Create your own path. Be your own version of awesome!

CHAPTER 22

Step into your power

Step into your power

There comes a time when you must let go and rise above all that's gone before. Shed your inhibitions and any limitations that have been holding you back. This is a necessary step, to build upon a solid foundation that can springboard you to the new level of success you wish to achieve.

Success connection

Surround yourself with people who share your vision for success. Choose a higher vibration group, where love exists from deep within. Let your energy explode in unison with those called to meet you on that higher plane. It's a place where like-minded souls can live and play in abundance, as they choose their paths of hidden treasures – one that only a few can find. This will help you maintain a steady path, along your journey toward success.

Be open

Be open to shifting your ideas and current state of mind, especially from negative to positive. Up-levelling is likely to involve some changes, which may not make sense to those around you at first. They will be necessary, however, to become the woman of your dreams. Change is inevitable, so, embrace it!

Write down your heart's desire

Tap into the reason behind why you want to achieve success, including the impact it will have on you and your loved ones. Write about what you want with wild abandon, expressing your deepest desires and wishes. You hold the keys to success within you. Allow yourself to dream a little bigger, shine much brighter and believe that you can be, do and achieve whatever you want in life.

Visualise success

Don't be afraid to aim high, towards the dizziest of heights! Visualise the success you want and really get into the finer details, including how it makes you feel. Try this short visualisation:

- Imagine waking up and being in your ideal life. Really 'feel' it into existence.

- Go through the specifics.

    o What does your home look like?

    o What will you eat for breakfast?

- Now, see yourself sitting outside, in a beautiful garden; notice a pathway that leads to the beach.

- Walk along the pathway and continue walking along the seashore. Feel the sand between your toes. Hear the waves lapping against the shore.

- Visualise yourself laughing, in pure delight.

    o Really explore the energy of this.

- What does success look and feel like, to you? Perhaps it's winning an award, speaking on a stage, getting across the

finish line of a marathon, or going on
an expedition, far away.

- o Really get into the feeling of it
     all and enjoy the experience.

- o Get excited about the possibility
     of your vision being your new
     reality. This will trigger a high
     vibration for success, welcoming
     all possibilities into existence.

- Open your eyes and reconnect to your
  present surroundings.

After you have done this exercise, you'll gain
a fresh outlook, with newfound optimism.
You might even have a twinkle in your eye, as
you smile to yourself with your inner
knowing that brighter things are to come. This
is where the fun begins!

Embody

Now, ask yourself, 'Who do I have to be to
achieve my dreams?' This is all about getting
into character and getting to know the highest
and brightest version of you. If you were free
from fear and limitations and could be

whoever you wanted to be, how would you act? If this seems far off, view a model of this person on someone else, to start with. What are her qualities and characteristics? How does she respond to challenges, situations and opportunities? What kind of clothes does she wear? What hairstyle does she have? Go into as much detail as possible.

Then, take a couple of minutes to think (and, ideally, also, write) about your own personal qualities. What do you love about yourself? What do you admire about you? What are your specific attributes? For instance, you may have a brilliant sense of humour, or find it easy to get on with other people, etc. Now, take the qualities that you love about you and combine them with the things you admire about your imaginary person. Clothe yourself in all of these wonderful qualities and look at yourself in the mirror. Feeling good?

Now you are ready to step into the shoes of the future you – that brighter, braver version of you. No more waiting; it's your time to shine and to be the rock star of your own gig. Polish up your star quality, so that you're

ready to shine bright and sparkle anew.
You're set to dazzle with your brilliance and
radiate your love. Ignite your passion!

Energy in presence

We all have energy within us, some of which
we give out to those around us. When you
feel down and out of sorts, you normally find
that your energy levels feel low. This can
cause you to want to withdraw and shun the
limelight. At other times, when your energy
level is much higher and more expansive, you
are more likely to feel happy and ready to
party! It's often at these moments that you feel
you can achieve anything you want to. The
high vibrational frequency that derives from
this energy is where the real magic happens!
By cultivating it, we are able to step into our
truest essence, giving us the capacity to be all
that we can be – and more.

Consciously being aware of energy levels
helps us to take control of our current state,
either increasing it or slowing it down, as
necessary. As an example, if you are feeling
down and find yourself in a low vibrational
state, try doing something to cheer you up.

Ask yourself, 'What can I do right now, to make me feel good?'.

Asking yourself a question, whether it's out loud or in your head, triggers the need to answer it. You'll find your mind immediately gets to work, in searching for responses! Once you have a couple of ideas, start doing them. This could be anything; it doesn't really matter what, exactly. You may want to play a favourite song, or draw a picture – or even go outside and plant a flower. Do what works for you! Afterwards, you'll find that, because you've done something different and altered your state of mind, you feel better. This then increases your energy level, giving you an instant boost. You can now switch on your positive energy and high vibrational frequency more often. The more you do it, the easier it becomes.

Now that you have control over your energy, you can have some fun with it and really feel it magnetise. For instance, when you walk down the road, feel your energy expanding around you. You could give it a colour – say gold, for example. Then, just imagine it getting bigger and bigger. This will inevitably impact those around you in a positive way, too. Then imagine this light becoming smaller and contracting. Once you get the hang of it, it can help you in many situations. Good examples are those times when you'd like to feel more confident, such as at a party, or when you're about to go on stage.

On the other hand, if you want to rest and chill out, practice slowing down and withdrawing your energy; try keeping it to yourself for a while, whilst you're recharging. Practising energy in presence can redefine who you are and make you more 'you'.

Love yourself so much that it makes you glow from the inside, full of vitality. Then your energy can better attract people who appreciate you. When you value yourself and feel that you are worthy of having the best in life, you'll attract more good vibes to you. You'll be able to magnetise all things good to you. Be magnetic in your presence!

You are blessed with a vision for a reason. You already have the ability to make things happen. You just have to believe this, do the work and keep the fire inside of you burning.

Let your presence be known to many and allow your heart to stay true to you. Follow your light and see where it takes you. Shine bright in your essence; it belongs to you. Light up the sky, because the world needs your light!

Leave behind a legacy. You were born for this moment. The life of your dreams is your birth right.

Go get it, Beautiful!

CHAPTER 23

Thrive

Your definition of success

Success can mean different things to different
people, find your definition of success and
decide what it means to you. You, alone, live
by your own definition. For one person, it
could mean climbing a mountain; for another
it could be finishing off a school project with
their child. No two people are alike and their
versions of success are just as distinct from
one another.

While climbing the corporate ladder of
success, I learnt that – for me – something was
missing. This eventually affected my health
and resulted in requiring regular time off; my
periods of absence were often due to feeling
unwell. In my quest to find out why this was
happening, I embarked on my personal
spiritual path, where I experimented with
affirmations, crystals and aromatherapy. As I

strove to find the missing pieces of the puzzle, my intuition sharpened. It did so to the point that I just knew something wasn't right – and that things would have to change before my life could get better (or, perhaps I should say, before *I* could get better).

Let go

That was when I learnt to let go of the things that no longer served me. They included both the corporate world and my lifestyle. It wasn't an easy decision to make because, from the outside looking in, I had it all! Yet, something didn't feel quite right, so I went with my gut instinct and took a risk. This was so unlike me. I was a banker, after all; risk-taking was not really in my vocabulary. But this feeling was so strong, it almost had a sense of urgency about it. So, I simply had to take notice! Once I did, there was no looking back. And, you know what? It felt so good! It felt like a whole weight had been lifted from my shoulders. I felt able to breathe again, finally (and, for an asthmatic, that was quite a big deal!)

I do remember some people thinking I was crazy, because I had nothing planned. There was no job set-up to go to. But I knew, in my heart of heart's, that it was the right move. I was doing what felt right for me and that felt amazing! It was possibly selfish, too, but nevertheless still felt AMAZING.

Ask yourself, now, when was the last time you felt so amazing – when you did something that was just right for you? If you haven't done so already, I suggest you give it a go! It'll give you such a boost, uplifting your soul in ways you never thought possible. Go on – I dare you!

Take a risk, now and then

The reason for sharing my story with you is to underline that we need to be able to take risks, every so often, in order to truly thrive. So, find the risk-taker within you – the gambler and go-getter, who won't take, 'No', for an answer. I know she's somewhere inside you. If you care to seek her out, I promise you'll find her. We all have her in us. It's just a case of having the courage and determination to look hard enough to access

213

her. I'm not going to lie; this takes guts. But, you know what? You can do it! I'm sure of this and believe in you; now it's your turn. Be a mover and shaker. Be a conversation-starter – and a dream maker.

Let your dreams become more than just, 'Some day…'

They deserve better, and you deserve more.

On the edge of my seat

I always had the habit of sitting on the edge of my seat. It was as if I was afraid to be at ease and relax completely. I was constantly, ready, to get up and go.

I now realise that this was a sign of restlessness to do with my hunger for success; not everyone else's version of success, only mine. Instead of just sitting back and dreaming, I knew I had to play my part – I had to take action.

Action bridges the gap

I'm not a sit-back-and-do-nothing kind of girl. I take action, without the need to talk about it, until the task is done! I do this, because I know that action bridges the gap between the dream and reality.

So, go and do what you are meant to do, and get on with it until your task is completed. Then, hold your head up high and stand proud, in the knowledge that you saw it through until the end.

You're in this for the long haul. A sprint never wins the final game, so, conserve your emotional and physical energy. Do less and *be* more. Think of quality over quantity. A lot of stress comes from trying to do too many things. Simplify your life and feel the pressure drop off. You are not a machine! Work at a steady and consistent pace, then release any pent-up passion just before you see the goal in sight. Prepare for a battle that requires strength, courage and perseverance, but – above all – also, love for yourself and others, to see you through until the end.

Don't be afraid

Don't be afraid to thrive. You don't always have to go through tough times to grow.

Good times, including those in which you have the most success, can help you grow, too. Even though stepping out of your comfort zone may seem nerve-wracking, it can also uncover qualities you never realised you had. We are all continuously learning, even about ourselves.

Entering a new stage of life requires patience, endurance and understanding, but those are equally your rewards. You can't buy them; they're gifts to be treasured. Embrace new experiences with love, and welcome those miracles of wonder into your life with open arms.

What are you looking forward to next?

Your presence

Keep a reminder of your greatest qualities, whether this means writing them down to read in future, or recording spoken 'notes' of them, which you can play back to yourself. Doing so at regular intervals will help you tap into what you are all about, to help you preserve your inner strength. It can serve as a memory point, whenever you're feeling 'less than', or down about something. While not everything will always go to plan, if you can remember all the good things about you, and what makes you tick, then the bad stuff will more likely bounce off you. This helps build resilience. It can also mean you are less worried about trying out new things, because you know what you are made of – and that you have the ability to bounce back with ease.

Realise who you are. Build a firm foundation, so that you can stand strong in your presence, instead of hesitating. Stay driven, in your pursuit for success. Be purposeful in your approach and walk like you are going places – like you really mean it! Know that every step has an intention. You are not a drifter without rhyme or reason. You are the queen of your own life, so, act like one! Remember the greatness in you. Be proud of yourself. Speak with the confidence and assurance that you have something of value to say. Be proud of all that you have accomplished. No one else can cheer you on like you can!

Be charming; be poised and graceful in your attitude. Set your elegance in motion and let confidence and charisma ooze out of every pore. Be filled with vitality, as you strive for optimum performance and ever-expanding success, even as you bask in your present state. You'll never have this moment again, so, 'wow' your now!

Be a magnet of success

You are an expression of art, in its full glory. Elevate your mindset, as part of your growth. Be aware of your magnificence; let it expand for the world to see. Keep hold of your sense of adventure, as you explore new horizons. Stay ever the opportunist, as you become bolder. Leave something to be remembered by; an essence of mystery in your wake. Be a magnet of success and let the trail of success follow your every move.

Own yourself, as you step forward in strength and passion – for you were born for greatness. If you're to take anything away from this book, remember this: value yourself and keep on celebrating you!

CONCLUSION

You are not here to merely survive. You are here to thrive, and to enjoy this wonderful journey of life.

So, go and be that mover and shaker. Be the go-getter and star-maker, who puts you at the centre of the show.

You deserve to be held in high regard, respected for your ambition and admired for your talents.

I know there is more to you than meets the eye – and, deep down, so do you. Give yourself the chance to show just what you're made of. In a world full of shadows, be the light. In a story filled with, 'Perhaps' and, 'Maybe', be the, 'Oh yes!' and 'Watch me!'

Let your passion be like rocket fuel, in your desire for success.

Look up at the night sky and fill it with starlight and sparkles, as you soar into your grand vision, magnified with wonder and surprise.

She is calling, beckoning you into action; can you hear her? Even better, can you *feel* her? Unleash the superstar within you and be the woman of wonder you've always wanted to be. You were born for this very moment.

Go get it, Beautiful.

After all is said and done, you deserve to feel amazing and thrive.

Cheers, to your brilliance!

The best is yet to come...

SHARE THE LOVE

Have you found this book helpful?

If so, please tell someone about it by leaving a review.

You could help make a difference to someone else's life.

Want to keep in touch?

Join my Author Friends List & receive your Free digital gift at:

pamelasommers.com

ACKNOWLEDGEMENTS

Thank you to my editor, Diana McMahon Collis, for your support and encouragement.

To you, my reader: I thank you for taking the time to read this book,

which I wrote especially for you.

I wish you a life full of love and happiness,

may blessings follow, wherever you go.

THANK YOU

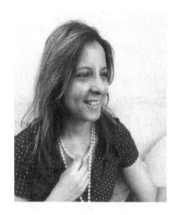

ABOUT THE AUTHOR

Pamela Sommers is an award-winning author of the bestsellers, *Life lessons from a 40 Something...: For The Best Start In Life*, *Building Castles In The Sky: How To Make Your Dreams Come True* and *Fabulously You: Live a Life You Love*. She has been featured in a number of publications, including *Success, House of Coco,* and *Spotlight* magazines, as well as *The Independent, Metro, and Belfast Telegraph*. Her tips and advice for entrepreneurs have also graced the *HuffPost, Thrive Global* and *LadyBossBlogger* blogs.

She is the Founder of *SommerSparkle*, an international, multi-award-winning, online boutique that provides beautiful jewellery & accessories for special occasions. Several pieces have been showcased in magazines, such as *British Vogue*.

Pamela is passionate about inspiring others to make their dreams come true. She enjoys horse-riding and loves to dance and listen to music. She currently lives in London, England with her fiancé and son.

You can find her online at

pamelasommers.com

www.instagram.com/pamela.sommers

www.facebook.com/PamelaSommersOfficial

sommersparkle.com

READ MORE FROM THE AUTHOR...

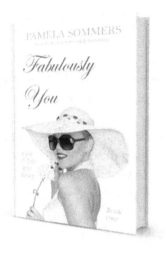

Fabulously You:

Live a Life You Love

(Book One)

Pamela's bestselling, personal growth book
helps you to reconnect and re-discover

yourself. It empowers you to live a life that's true to you.

Here's what people are saying about it:

'For those who are fearful of the future, this is one to read'

'I also liked the author's emphasis on looking after yourself, bringing love, kindness and tenderness back into our lives and, most importantly, being true to ourselves.'

'A toolkit for life filled with happy delights'

'Ms. Sommers hits the nail right on the head with her life observations and positive advice. Each chapter is devoted to a specific "life lesson" that offers encouragement and inspiration to be the very best version of yourself you can be. I recommend this book for anyone interested in a positive attitude adjustment or anyone looking for ways to change their outlook on life.'

'Sunshine in a book, a go-to for happy living.'

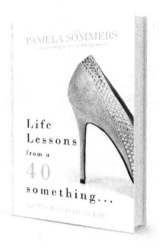

Life Lessons from a 40 something... :

For The Best Start In Life

Pamela's award-winning, bestselling, self-improvement book is filled with big-hearted advice, to empower and inspire you to go for your dreams—regardless of your current circumstances. It is based on her own life.

229

Here's what people are saying about it:

'An easy read and truly inspirational, even life changing.'

'This book imparts lessons, with each chapter delivering its own lesson theme, such as "Don't compare yourself to others," etc. Some include how the author came to learn these lessons, and most include why they are important.'

'As a therapist, these are all the same lessons that I strive to teach my clients so that may live healthy lives that are true to their values and selves. There is great wisdom in this book, and I wish I had read it when I was about fifteen. You will be glad you picked it up, and hopefully you will share it, too.'

'Sound advice written in an informal manner from a personal perspective. There are things in this book that just reading the words alone will have a massive impact on a person. Realising you in yourself are enough can go a long way. For me, this book is about trusting who you are, even if you're not quite sure who that is. After all, you always change and

grow… Easily accessible, not preachy, and very insightful.'

'Big-hearted advice from a wise lady. This is a warm and useful book that I would recommend to anyone from the age of 16 to 40. It covers all the issues that make someone a happy, thriving, successful member of society – from love relationships to being confident in the workplace to how to look great. The author writes clearly in a style that can be understood and applied by any age group, and she gives examples of exercises you can use to implement the ideas she suggests…The new material you do take away will help you live a happier, more fulfilled life.'

'Life Lessons is a book that I wish I would have read years ago. It gives you much-needed wisdom to conquer all the obstacles that you will experience in life, as well as giving you sound advice for getting through the highs and lows. This is a book that should be read by teenagers and 20 somethings, to avoid any quarter-life crisis. As I knock on the door of 40, these are lessons that I still can apply.'

'Although geared toward teenagers and young adults, "Life Lessons from a 40 something" has all sorts of good advice applicable for all

231

ages, even those of us who are 40 something, as well. A pleasant read, full of Ms. Sommers personal experiences and the lessons she learned over the years.'- The International Review of Books

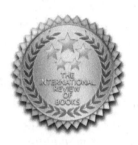

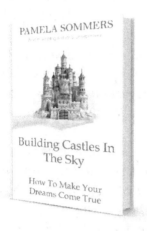

Building Castles In The Sky :

How To Make Your Dreams Come True

Pamela's bestselling, personal growth book is filled with spiritual secrets for success, to help make your dreams come true.

Here's what people are saying about it:

'An uplifting and helpful book, for all those wishing to become the best version of themselves.'

'I really enjoyed reading this positive and uplifting self-help book. I plan to put her suggestions into practice. I am looking forward to positive change.'

'This book is easy to follow and understand. I recommend it to anyone looking to improve their life. It is confidence-inspiring for any age reader. I commend the author for sharing these valuable insights into life and how to make it better.'

'Wonderful - It's an inspiring guide to those seeking calm and peace in a chaotic world. I read it as part of my therapy for social anxiety, and I will definitely be recommending it to others.'

'There are some excellent examples of behaviour (I found myself in there a number of times) and a heap of advice and tips on how to changes your thoughts and get back on track. An easy read, highly recommended.'

'If only I had read her book earlier, because my ride would definitely have been smoother and easier with her help!'

'The author's references to Biblical times and scriptures from the Bible bring relevance to Christians. "God wants us to experience all the good things in life." The author shares personal stories of her journey and a roadmap with tools for 'building castles in the sky', guiding you through the steps you will need to take, in an easy-to- understand writing style.'

Available at leading book retailers.

NOTES

NOTES

CPSIA information can be obtained
at www.ICGtesting.com
Printed in the USA
BVHW091149300421
606207BV00002B/205

9 781916 358751